"Knowing is not enough; we must apply.
Willing is not enough; we must do."
—Goethe

INSTITUTE OF MEDICINE
OF THE NATIONAL ACADEMIES

Advising the Nation. Improving Health.

THE NATIONAL ACADEMIES

Advisers to the Nation on Science, Engineering, and Medicine

The **National Academy of Sciences** is a private, nonprofit, self-perpetuating society of distinguished scholars engaged in scientific and engineering research, dedicated to the furtherance of science and technology and to their use for the general welfare. Upon the authority of the charter granted to it by the Congress in 1863, the Academy has a mandate that requires it to advise the federal government on scientific and technical matters. Dr. Ralph J. Cicerone is president of the National Academy of Sciences.

The **National Academy of Engineering** was established in 1964, under the charter of the National Academy of Sciences, as a parallel organization of outstanding engineers. It is autonomous in its administration and in the selection of its members, sharing with the National Academy of Sciences the responsibility for advising the federal government. The National Academy of Engineering also sponsors engineering programs aimed at meeting national needs, encourages education and research, and recognizes the superior achievements of engineers. Dr. Charles M. Vest is president of the National Academy of Engineering.

The **Institute of Medicine** was established in 1970 by the National Academy of Sciences to secure the services of eminent members of appropriate professions in the examination of policy matters pertaining to the health of the public. The Institute acts under the responsibility given to the National Academy of Sciences by its congressional charter to be an adviser to the federal government and, upon its own initiative, to identify issues of medical care, research, and education. Dr. Harvey V. Fineberg is president of the Institute of Medicine.

The **National Research Council** was organized by the National Academy of Sciences in 1916 to associate the broad community of science and technology with the Academy's purposes of furthering knowledge and advising the federal government. Functioning in accordance with general policies determined by the Academy, the Council has become the principal operating agency of both the National Academy of Sciences and the National Academy of Engineering in providing services to the government, the public, and the scientific and engineering communities. The Council is administered jointly by both Academies and the Institute of Medicine. Dr. Ralph J. Cicerone and Dr. Charles M. Vest are chair and vice chair, respectively, of the National Research Council.

www.national-academies.org

MILITARY MEDICAL ETHICS

ISSUES REGARDING DUAL LOYALTIES

Workshop Summary

Neil E. Weisfeld, Victoria D. Weisfeld, and Catharyn T. Liverman,
Rapporteurs

Board on Health Sciences Policy

INSTITUTE OF MEDICINE
OF THE NATIONAL ACADEMIES

THE NATIONAL ACADEMIES PRESS
Washington, D.C.
www.nap.edu

THE NATIONAL ACADEMIES PRESS • 500 Fifth Street, N.W. • Washington, DC 20001

NOTICE: The project that is the subject of this report was approved by the Governing Board of the National Research Council, whose members are drawn from the councils of the National Academy of Sciences, the National Academy of Engineering, and the Institute of Medicine. The members of the committee responsible for the report were chosen for their special competences and with regard for appropriate balance.

This project was supported by Award No. W81XWH-07-F-0541 between the National Academy of Sciences and the U.S. Department of Defense through Experient, Inc., and by a grant from The Greenwall Foundation.

International Standard Book Number-13: 978-0-309-12663-2
International Standard Book Number-10: 0-309-12663-0

Additional copies of this report are available from the National Academies Press, 500 Fifth Street, N.W., Lockbox 285, Washington, DC 20055; (800) 624-6242 or (202) 334-3313 (in the Washington metropolitan area); Internet, http://www.nap.edu.

For more information about the Institute of Medicine, visit the IOM home page at: **www.iom.edu.**

Printed in the United States of America

Suggested citation: IOM (Institute of Medicine). 2009. *Military medical ethics: Issues regarding dual loyalties: Workshop summary.* Washington, DC: The National Academies Press.

WORKSHOP ON MILITARY MEDICAL ETHICS PLANNING COMMITTEE*

JAMES F. CHILDRESS (*Chair*), University of Virginia
SCOTT A. ALLEN, Brown University Medical School
PAUL S. APPELBAUM, Columbia University Medical Center
THOMAS E. BEAM, COL (retired), MC, U.S. Army
RICHARD J. BONNIE, University of Virginia
LONNIE BRISTOW, American Medical Association (retired)
LINDA EMANUEL, Northwestern University
EDMUND HOWE, Uniformed Services University of the Health Sciences
SANDRAL HULLETT, Cooper Green Hospital
M. E. BONNIE ROGERS, University of North Carolina, School of Public Health, Chapel Hill

Adviser to the Planning Committee
ELENA O. NIGHTINGALE, IOM Scholar-in-Residence

Study Staff
CATHARYN T. LIVERMAN, Study Director
FRANKLIN BRANCH, Research Associate
JUDY ESTEP, Program Associate
ANDREW M. POPE, Director, Board on Health Sciences Policy
FREDERICK ERDTMANN, Director, Board on Military and Veterans Health
CAROL CORILLON, Director, Committee on Human Rights

*IOM planning committees are solely responsible for organizing the workshop, identifying topics, and choosing speakers. The responsibility for the published workshop summary rests with the workshop rapporteurs and the institution.

Independent Report Reviewers

This report has been reviewed in draft form by individuals chosen for their diverse perspectives and technical expertise, in accordance with procedures approved by the National Research Council's Report Review Committee. The purpose of this independent review is to provide candid and critical comments that will assist the institution in making its published report as sound as possible and to ensure that the report meets institutional standards for objectivity, evidence, and responsiveness to the study charge. The review comments and draft manuscript remain confidential to protect the integrity of the deliberative process. We wish to thank the following individuals for their review of this report:

George J. Annas, Department of Health Law, Bioethics and Human Rights, Boston University School of Public Health
Thomas E. Beam, U.S. Army (retired)
Lonnie R. Bristow, American Medical Association
Frederick M. Burkle, Harvard Humanitarian Initiative, Harvard University and Schools of Public Health and Medicine, Johns Hopkins University Medical Institutions, and U.S. Navy (retired)
Thomas C. Jefferson, Department of Clinical Investigation, Brooke Army Medical Center, U.S. Army
Elspeth Cameron Ritchie, Strategic Communication Directorate, Army Medical Department
Stephen Olufemi Sodeke, Tuskegee University National Center for Bioethics in Research & Health Care

Although the reviewers listed above have provided many constructive comments and suggestions, they did not see the final draft of the report before its release. The review of this report was overseen by **Christine K. Cassel,** American Board of Internal Medicine. Appointed by the Institute of Medicine, she was responsible for making certain that an independent examination of this report was carried out in accordance with institutional procedures and that all review comments were carefully considered. Responsibility for the final content of this report rests entirely with the authoring committee and the institution.

Preface

In finding common ground on the ethics of health care, the discussions held during this workshop highlighted the fact that military health professionals are not alone in facing dual loyalties—responsibilities to two or more entities. Corporate occupational health professionals deal with the push and pull of employers, workers, and unions. Sports medicine professionals from trainers to team physicians face questions and quandaries posed by players, parents, coaches, and administrators. Health professionals in correctional facilities work on matters of concern to the inmates and to management. As the workshop participants examined these issues and addressed them in light of two case studies specific to military health professionals, the similarities and differences with situations in the civilian sector pointed to the need for greater sharing of ideas across sectors as well as for increased transparency to the extent feasible consistent with national security concerns.

Although the ethical issues faced by the military in situations in Abu Ghraib and Guantanamo were a backdrop of this workshop, these discussions looked forward at ways to continue to improve military training, policy, and structure to better support ethical decisions by military health professionals.

Throughout the exchange of diverse perspectives and expertise, it became clear that the military experience can inform and be informed by ethical dilemmas faced in other health care settings. What was striking was the breath and depth of common ground. The paramount value of the patient–provider relationship was recognized, but many questions remain about how best to address other responsibilities as well as the realities of different organizational structures and cultures.

It was a privilege to chair this Institute of Medicine workshop. Planning committee members and workshop speakers were diligent in their thorough preparation, thoughtful presentations, and considered comments. In addition, workshop participants raised insightful questions and provided further information that added to the open dialogue.

The groundwork for this workshop was provided through the insightful discussions of the National Academies' Committee on Human Rights, the IOM Board on Military and Veterans Health, and the IOM Board on Health Sciences Policy.

The military services, as with other organizations, will continue to benefit from ongoing discourse about common and distinctive ethical quandaries.

James F. Childress, *Chair*
Planning Committee

Contents

SUMMARY[1]

This report summarizes the proceedings of a one-day workshop, "Military Medical Ethics: Issues Regarding Dual Loyalties," convened by the Institute of Medicine on September 8, 2008. The purpose of the workshop was to examine ethical challenges for physicians and other health professionals serving in the military that arise from conflicts between their responsibilities to patients and their duties as military officers. Dual loyalties exist in many medical fields, from occupational health to public health. Military health professionals, as all health professionals, are ethically responsible for their patients' well-being. In some situations, however, military health professionals can face ethical tensions between responsibilities to individual patients and responsibilities to military operations.

Indeed, everyone has conflicting allegiances, partly as a matter of choice and partly as a matter of chance. Because dual loyalties involve multiple responsibilities that are not usually laid out in parallel or made to reinforce each other, moments of tension arise between them. The workshop proceeded from the premise that such conflicts are best brought to light and discussed by military and civilian leaders rather than relegated to individuals to cope with them alone in situations of stress.

---

[1]The planning committee's role was limited to planning the workshop, and the workshop summary has been prepared by the workshop rapporteurs as a factual summary of what occurred at the workshop.

To illustrate how dual loyalties can influence decisions of U.S. military health care providers, two case studies were presented based on circumstances that a provider might encounter in the military setting. Decisions regarding whether to return an injured servicemember to duty after a closed head injury, despite the risk of greater harm, offered the situations for the first case study. Return-to-duty decisions are replete with unintended consequences, ranging from impacts on a soldier's (or disabled veteran's) compensation to effects on the morale and overall performance of the individual and the fighting unit. One consideration in these decisions is that there are opportunities in military service to return a servicemember to duty on a trial basis with the potential for change of duty or evacuation as needed.

Dual loyalty situations, with some relevant similarities, exist in occupational medicine and sports medicine. In occupational medicine, particularly in small corporations, where the physician or nurse reports directly to corporate executives, an injured employee's desire to return to work in order to obtain full benefits may conflict with corporate productivity goals. In sports medicine, a triad of decision makers—physician, coach, and athlete—typically make a joint decision, based on a full assessment of risks and benefits offered by the physician.

Treating detainees in ethically charged circumstances, such as a hunger strike, provided the situations for the second case study. International declarations require physicians to respect the autonomy of hunger strikers, who may have no other recourse to protest conditions of confinement. The U.S. Department of Defense (DoD) policy of beneficence would permit force-feeding to save a prisoner's life. In the civilian world, physicians working in correctional facilities have found it important to earn prisoners' trust and to use that trust to defuse potential crises by seeking alternatives, such as transferring the striking prisoner to another health facility.

The hunger strike case study showed that two factors are fundamentally important in ethical decision making: the presence of organizational resources to help physicians manage ethical quandaries without having to resort to heroic tactics, and the recognition of the particular and often distinctive circumstances of each case. At times there is a cultural component to ethical issues involving hunger strikers. For example, Islamic scholars have advised that hunger-striking to the point of impending death is not a valid action in their faith, so long as detainees are allowed to perform their religious duties.

Addressing the need for training in medical ethics can involve a range of approaches. At the Uniformed Services University of the Health Sciences, medical ethics is an essential element of the core curriculum and encompasses varied teaching methods, including inviting speakers to discuss their experiences, case study discussions, and field practice exercises. Continuing education of health professionals offers ongoing opportunities to learn from interdisciplinary perspectives. Training outside the classroom in a real-world situation, such as aboard a naval hospital ship on a humanitarian mission, offers teachable moments for addressing ethical dilemmas. Innovative approaches for enhancing ethics training are being tried in various contexts. For example, at Northwestern University, training in ethical issues in palliative medicine includes interdisciplinary hospital rounds, interactions with patients in nonclinical settings, and instruction focused on real patients and their life experiences—sometimes presented through videotaped interviews.

Organizational values and behavior strongly influence adherence to ethical principles. In the military, the commander sets the tone, as does his or her counterpart in civilian senior management. A just organization exhibits ethical awareness, judgment, and motivation and implements ethical standards. A step that organizations can take to strengthen their ethical infrastructure is to establish an ombudsperson's office to investigate individual complaints and report findings in the aggregate, without personal identifiers. Ensuring that organizations act ethically requires involving staff at many levels, along with organizational feedback, deliberation, organized advocacy, and appropriate checks and balances, some of which may be external to the organization.

Within the military services, primary responsibility to the patient should prevail in nearly all circumstances. This workshop focused on situations in which ethical conflicts arise because of dual loyalties. Workshop participants emphasized several points:

- Dual loyalty situations can occur in military medicine, although in most routine aspects of health care, military medicine is similar to civilian medicine.
- Models used in occupational medicine, sports medicine, and prison medicine, among others, can be informative in considering ways to address ethical issues in military medicine.
- Some important differences exist between international declarations and DoD health policies regarding hunger strikes. The two views cannot easily be reconciled in the abstract, but, in many

situations, consideration of individual circumstances could lead to the same result under either approach.

- Ethical considerations relevant to military medicine include parity, elasticity, and *primum non nocere.*[2] Transparency of policies and practices should be paramount, except in those situations when legitimate security concerns require setting limits on the disclosure of information.
- Patient trust in health care professionals is vital for a productive provider–patient relationship, yet sometimes difficult to engender in circumstances of dual loyalty.
- Ethical decision making requires more than prioritizing separate principles, such as autonomy and beneficence. The ethical principles must be recognized, specified, and balanced in practical ways that build trust and preserve the dignity of each person.

INTRODUCTION

- Are there situations in which military medical ethics differ from the ethics of a civilian medical practice? If so, how do the obligations of a military officer and a military health professional differ?
- What other models could be used to examine these conflicts (e.g., occupational health)?
- How do existing national and international standards of medical ethics apply to military physicians, and what is their relationship to national and international law?
- What are the ethical principles that guide medical practice for military physicians? Do these principles differ from those of the broader medical community?

These four central questions were the starting point for discussion at an all-day workshop, "Military Medical Ethics: Issues Regarding Dual Loyalties," conducted by the Institute of Medicine (IOM) of the National Academies on September 8, 2008. Jointly sponsored by the Office of the Assistant Secretary of Defense for Health Affairs and the Greenwall

[2]In this context, *parity* refers to equality in treating patients, *elasticity* refers to flexibility in implementing policies, and *primum non nocere* is the historic principle of "first, do no harm."

Foundation, the workshop was held at the National Academies building in Washington, DC. Seventy-three registered participants, representing diverse perspectives from academic, military, business, human rights, and health professions, contributed to the discussion.

The workshop was not intended to generate firm rules or a prescription for change; rather, it was intended to serve as a forum for discussion of the ethical challenges for physicians and other health professionals serving in the military—ethical challenges that sometimes arise from conflicts between their responsibilities to patients and their duties as military officers. A planning committee of 10 members, assisted by IOM staff, designed the workshop to that end. The committee's role was limited to determining the format, setting the agenda, and choosing speakers, session moderators, topics, background readings, and two case studies to be used in the discussion. This report was prepared by the rapporteurs as a factual summary of the workshop discussion; it consolidates the views of the individual participants but is not intended to reflect a consensus of those attending.

Background materials provided for the workshop defined dual loyalty situations (also termed *mixed agency*) as those in which health professionals are obligated to fulfill multiple roles, sometimes resulting in ethical tensions between the roles (Beam and Sparacino, 2003; Appendix A).

The workshop focused on two specific situations in which military health professionals may face ethical conflicts because of dual loyalties—decisions regarding returning servicemembers to duty following an injury or health concern and decisions regarding the care of hunger strikers. The military is only one of many environments that involve dual loyalties. Selected others include

- *occupational health,* where a physician serves both patients and employers;
- *infectious disease or mental health practice,* where a clinician may have to balance the patient's interests and demands against those of the patient's family, sexual partners, or other individuals at potential risk of harm by the patient (Johnson et al., 2006);
- *sports medicine,* where a physician or athletic trainer serves both the athlete and a sports organization or team;
- *forensic medicine,* where a physician consultant serves the court but also has some responsibilities to the individual being examined (Strasburger et al., 1997); and

- *public health practice,* where a community's interest in immunizations or quarantine may conflict with an individual's interest, religious conviction, or preference.

It is difficult for ethical arbiters and instructors to articulate the precise ethical obligations of physicians in such varied, complex, and pressured situations. However, once articulated in the abstract, these obligations also must be effectively imparted to, and internalized by, current and future physicians likely to face such dilemmas. Educational models for medical ethics exist in several settings, such as military medical education, training in end-of-life care, and preparation of medical ombudspersons.

TOWARD A FRAMEWORK FOR RESOLVING DUAL LOYALTIES

The workshop discussion commenced with a description of its context. The immediate and vital task in resolving dual loyalties is to lay out the difficulties. IOM President Harvey Fineberg observed, "Every one of us in our lives takes on different roles, some of them by chance, and some by choice." Legal contracts, moral compacts, and other allegiances affect these relationships and responsibilities. Volunteers in the U.S. military service accept profound responsibilities—on oath[3]—but often these responsibilities are not clearly laid out in parallel or made to reinforce each other. As a result, said Fineberg, "moments of tension" arise, morally and in other ways. He offered as an "underlying premise" of the workshop the belief that these difficult issues do not benefit from being ignored or secretly managed or considered to be implicit. Rather, discussions such as those conducted during this workshop "can provide an opportunity for reconciliation, for clarity, for decision making that will be based on ethical principles and guided by the realities" in carrying out the dual roles of health professional and military officer.

---

[3]The oath of office of military officers is similar to oaths taken by civilian officials: "I . . . do solemnly swear (or affirm) that I will support and defend the Constitution of the United States against all enemies, foreign or domestic; that I will bear true faith and allegiance to the same; that I take this obligation freely, without any mental reservations or purpose of evasion; and that I will well and faithfully discharge the duties of the office upon which I am about to enter, so help me God" (U.S. Army, 2004).

Negotiating ethical issues in military medicine is not simply a matter of implementing previously agreed-upon principles. Applying these principles in real-world situations involves health professionals making practical judgments in complex circumstances. Joseph Kelley, Deputy Assistant Secretary of Defense for Clinical and Program Policy, observed that issues of medical ethics in the military often correspond to contentious issues in civilian medical practice. For example, the military decision about return to duty is similar to the decision in sports medicine about keeping a player in a game, and the military physician's need to recognize organizational interests is similar to the pressure exerted on the managed care physician to deny expensive medical procedures that are not cost-effective. Opportunities exist to improve the training of both military and civilian health professionals in working through these complex issues.

Facing dual loyalties is nothing new for physicians and other health professionals; these issues have a history in military and other contexts and have often evoked vigorous and even heated discussion. Workshop Planning Committee Chair James F. Childress, Director of the University of Virginia Institute for Practical Ethics and Public Life, observed that the workshop discussion is designed to bring varied perspectives together to focus on opportunities for improving policy, practice, training, and individual and organizational decision making relevant to these types of ethical dilemmas. Childress noted that the intent of the workshop is not to investigate past allegations. In addressing dual loyalty, Childress said, the workshop will discuss which ethical principles are involved, whether these principles must be prioritized, what guidance exists and what needs to be developed, and who the ultimate decision makers are as well as how the training and other support they need will be provided. Ethically defining and balancing multiple role responsibilities and divided loyalties are the challenges for the discussion and for future action.

ETHICAL DECISION MAKING: RETURN TO DUTY

The participants in the first panel discussion considered a case study of ethical challenges to physicians charged with recommending whether to return a sick or injured servicemember to combat (or other fields of duty) (Box 1). The case study, involving a traumatic brain injury and risk of posttraumatic stress disorder (PTSD), included two situations that differed in whether the soldier wished to return to combat.

BOX 1

Case Study 1
Return to Duty: Ethical Issues for Military Health Professionals

A U.S. soldier suffers injuries from the explosion of an improvised explosive device. Injuries include closed-head injury resulting in loss of consciousness. After six weeks of treatment, the soldier is medically stable and functional, though he continues to complain of fatigue, disturbed sleep, and daily headaches. It is likely that he would be at higher risk for more severe impairment and PTSD if he were to suffer another similar explosion resulting in further traumatic brain injury.

Situation 1: The soldier is eager to return to the front lines and even when provided with the information on potential detrimental health consequences is willing to take his chances and return to his unit. The soldier is very insistent that he understands the risks and feels that the best way to resume his life is to return to his unit. His commanding officers express the strong need for his expertise and experience but do not exert any pressure to return the soldier to his former patrolling duties.

Situation 2: The soldier does not want to return to his patrolling duties and asks for reassignment. The physician suspects that the soldier may be exaggerating the symptoms that he is experiencing, though clearly considerable residual effects remain. However, personnel levels are low, with replacements several months down the road. Soldiers with his level of experience are desperately needed for upcoming missions, and there is strong pressure from the chain of command on the treating physician to sign off and return the soldier to his patrolling duties.

Considerations:

- What principles are in conflict?
- What guides the clinician in approaching each situation?
- What about the setting makes this situation different from civilian settings? Are the differences enough to warrant a separate rule?
- Who is the ultimate decision maker regarding decisions on return to the battlefront?
- What mechanisms or resources would help the health professional in resolving this conflict?

Military Considerations

The concept of fitness for duty incorporates the health of the individual and the overall health of the force. Even the health of the individual involves a multifaceted set of ethical factors. Colonel Elspeth Cameron Ritchie, Medical Director for Strategic Communication in the Army Medical Department, noted an increased emphasis in military medicine in recent years on patient education, prevention, and early diagnosis. The commander has the final call regarding return to duty, said Ritchie, but usually relies on physician recommendations, particularly when there is a recommendation for a medical evaluation board.

Data on decisions regarding return to duty are difficult to obtain because most communication has occurred through a paper medical profile that conveys health status and treatment information from the physician to the commander. As electronic medical records become more widespread, these data will become more accessible.

As a psychiatrist, Ritchie focused on behavioral health while noting similar issues for other medical fields. She outlined several key factors taken into account in return-to-duty decisions. In 2006 the DoD Office of Health Affairs developed standards for all military services requiring that deployed servicemembers meet military retention standards in order to be deployed and requiring a pattern of stability for three months for specific behavioral health diagnoses. A waiver process is available. Ritchie said that to date, 88 waivers have been requested with 22 of those disapproved. Determining the level of impairment for some psychiatric conditions can be challenging, given the potential impact of working in the operational theater. Decisions regarding acceptable medications for deployment (DoD, 2006a) have been made more complex by use of newer medications for some psychiatric conditions that may provide greater long-term stability when used in low doses. Although servicemembers on permanent antipsychotic regimens have been prohibited by policy from being returned to duty, newer medications, such as quetiapine, may provide long-term stability when used in low doses for treatment of symptoms associated with psychiatric conditions.

Other factors that affect return-to-duty decisions include access to treatment. Improved access to more sophisticated health care services now exists for PTSD and other mental health problems in mature theaters of operations, such as parts of Iraq. Further, return-to-duty decisions can include returning the servicemember to duty on a trial basis, with the potential for change of duty or evacuation as needed. Ritchie noted that the number of psychiatric casualties suffered by U.S. troops has not gone down and that there have been 20 to 40 evacuations per month for psychiatric reasons throughout the course of the war.

Return-to-duty decisions are fraught with the potential for unintended consequences. For example, a decision not to return a servicemember to duty can, in some cases, result in an administrative separation without disability compensation. And, for some patients, isolation from the soldier's usual environment can prove harmful emotionally. A decision to remove a soldier from harm's way for mental health reasons can potentially stigmatize the soldier.

In addressing the two situations of the case study, Ritchie commented that motivated soldiers who use the resources available for assessment and treatment have options available to return to duty at the pace needed or on a trial basis. Working with an unmotivated servicemember involves discussions between the commander and the physician with the possibility of temporary changes in job duty station or trial duty options.

Occupational Health Parallels

Occupational health professionals face ethical conflicts that may be instructive to their military counterparts. Several professional associations, including the American College of Occupational and Environmental Medicine and the International Commission on Occupational Health, have addressed dual loyalties—to the patient and to the employer—and call for putting responsibility to the patient first (ACOEM, 2008; ICOH, 2002). Large firms and other organizations usually try to return employees to work promptly, even if in another capacity. Myron C. Harrison, Senior Health Adviser at ExxonMobil Corporation, suggested that, by contrast, small organizations may need the employee in the same job and may not have the flexibility to assign individuals to new roles. Another difference is that in large organizations occupational medicine physicians typically report to another physician and therefore are somewhat insulated from business priorities, whereas their counterparts in smaller organizations often report to executives with bottom-line responsibilities who may be less tolerant of medical excuses. In smaller corporations, Harrison noted that the occupational health professional may also be more isolated. Occupational health often involves triaging and referring patients to specialists in the community. This involves early case management by working with the patient, family, and supervisor or management. External referrals are also used to assess the worker's ability to return to work, thus providing transparency and a greater measure of independence.

Harrison described ethical conflicts that typically involve competing "rights." Some matters, such as protections of employee confidentiality, are now prescribed by law and are dealt with through legal approaches. On ethical issues without legal mandates, Harrison noted that there are few if any algorithmic-type answers. As a touchstone, Harrison suggested that an act that *deceives* someone, whether the individual or the employer, probably is unethical. If no one—employee, manager, or labor union—is being deceived, then the matter probably is being handled transparently and on an ethical track. Harrison highlighted that safety-sensitive situations are managed very tightly with limitations on employee autonomy when third-party and plant safety is a concern.

Similar to medical profiles in the military (used for communicating medical treatment issues relevant to duty status between military physicians and commanders), communications by occupational health professionals to the worker's supervisor focus on conveying the limitations dictated by the patient's health status.

Regarding the case study, Harrison observed that the accuracy of the individual's description of symptoms often is doubted in cases such as those described in the second situation, when the individual does not wish to return to work, but is almost never doubted in the first situation, when the individual wishes to return. In a scenario similar to that of the motivated soldier, some occupational physicians would practice paternalism and would write a restriction from work, Harrison stated; relevant considerations include the magnitude of the risk and imminence of harm to the patient. In the situation of the unmotivated soldier, Harrison discussed temporarily placing the patient in a noncombat role while taking time to observe any progress.

Sports Medicine Parallels

Sports medicine offers other possible ethical parallels with military medicine. In competitive professional or interscholastic sports, a decision to return a sick or injured player to the field or court usually involves a triad of decision makers: the coach, the player, and the physician. Kurt P. Spindler, Professor of Orthopaedics and Rehabilitation at the Vanderbilt

University School of Medicine and head team physician for Vanderbilt's NCAA Division I varsity athletes, suggested that a military analog might consist of the commander, servicemember, and physician. Another similarity is the need to take into account the team's performance, which could be either strengthened or weakened by the player's return, depending in part on the availability of substitute players. A key difference between the sports and military venues is that an athlete has more autonomy than a member of the armed forces. Spindler noted differences between the levels of sports competition regarding the freedom of the athlete to choose the course of action. In high school, participation in sports is totally voluntary, and the physician acts as an adviser to the parents, student, and coach. In college the head physician makes the decision regarding playing status, which cannot be overruled by the coach or other collegiate officials. College students have a great deal of autonomy, although there are often scholarship and enrollment considerations. In professional sports, the players are under contract, and injuries involve worker compensation decisions and regulations.

As in occupational medicine, the sports medicine physician's primary responsibility is to the individual; in sports, this includes a duty to describe the risks and benefits of alternative treatments as well as the risks, and possible benefits, of continuing play. Transparency in decision making is essential.

Preventing a permanent injury is usually the main consideration. Other factors include

- the individual's freedom to choose;
- the specific role on the team and the extent to which the injury will affect the player's ability to perform (e.g., in football a hand injury is more harmful to a quarterback than to a lineman); and
- timing, as an individual might be appropriately returned after a delay but not immediately.

When an injury occurs, the sports medicine physician on the sidelines ideally takes the following steps: (1) defines the injury; (2) provides immediate treatment; (3) determines the risk; (4) assesses performance capability; (5) determines, in consultation with the coach, the benefit to the team; (6) discusses the alternatives with the coach and player; and (7) makes a final decision as part of the triad. The third step, risk assessment, is the pivotal task; it can lead to difficult decisions when, as often happens, there is a moderate risk, requiring close communication among the player, coach, and team.

Applying a sports context to the two situations outlined in the case study, Spindler stated that under the first scenario of a willing player and a clear risk of severe impairment such as a concussion, the player should not be returned immediately. Under the second scenario, if the patient does not have residual symptoms then the player can return, and the challenge is to regain the motivation to perform at a high level as part of the team.

Discussion

Comments focused first on the aptness of the analogies between problems arising in occupational and sports medicine and problems confronted in the military environment. Ritchie commented that a battlefield decision can, of course, be potentially far more consequential than an athletic field decision in terms of survival. Also, there may be more permanent consequences, because troops who leave for psychiatric or psychological reasons related to head injury or other concerns often do not return to the battlefield, and options can include early intervention and taking time to assess progress. The decision often does not involve weighing two "rights," she added, but weighing two wrongs, such as a pattern of being unmotivated against a pattern of putting too much pressure on troops. In addition, units with a high degree of cohesiveness generally manifest higher return rates. Lessons have been learned about rotating units rather than individuals in and out of the theater of operations to enhance those bonds. Harrison noted that a paternalistic, or "pseudo-paternalistic," decision (using the approach that the corporation knows what is best for the employee) not to return an individual to work in a corporation can be an easy way out of a dilemma; for example, many physicians permanently remove employees with low-back injuries despite the lack of medical evidence that such injuries tend to recur. Wages can be more important to the employee than a risk of future injury, so that a holistic view of health is needed with an emphasis on the individual's assessment and choice.

Organizational structure and information sharing can play an important role in return-to-duty decisions. For example, athletic trainers who are the first line of triage for sports injuries can be employed and supervised by the medical team—the ideal scenario—or they can be employed by the athletic department, where there is the potential for more pressures from the coaching staff and others. In the military, information sharing about medical conditions is limited to providing commanders with the information they need to know for job status and functional assessment. Ritchie noted that the medical profiles provided to commanders focus on what the soldier can or cannot do and on any problems that affect readiness to meet job demands.

Regarding psychiatric issues in the military, session moderator Paul S. Appelbaum from Columbia University Medical Center commented that the Army Medical Corps' rapid triage efforts to address issues close to the battlefield in World War II reduced long-term psychiatric morbidity and that lessons learned from those efforts launched the community psychiatry movement. Ritchie noted that until recently a servicemember's psychiatric history could negatively affect his or her security clearance. However, the policy of asking about seeking psychiatric counseling (the Question 21 issue on the government security clearance form) was relaxed in recent years—partly to improve PTSD diagnosis and treatment—by exempting combat-related psychiatric encounters from the grounds for reducing or revoking security clearances.

Discussion focused on the extent of patient autonomy in the military as compared with other situations. Ritchie noted that, with exceptions such as mandatory immunizations, military servicemembers have a great deal of influence over their own health care. Communication among the patient, health professional, and commander can be important in identifying problems that may have an impact on performing a specific job. An important consideration is the commander's responsibility for the health of all members of the unit. This can lead in many cases to decisions promoting and accommodating the individual's health but, in a few other cases, to decisions that give greater weight to the unit's interests. Differences between the military services were noted: In the Navy, for example, the captain of a ship at sea has responsibility for the life and health of all aboard and would be involved in major medical decisions.

Harrison noted similar issues in the private sector, including mandating that employees undertake chemoprophylaxis for malaria if they are working in areas where the disease is endemic. The corporation, in this case, followed up by monitoring employees through urine testing for the medication metabolites. A member of the audience raised a similar example—the requirement for school children to be immunized for specific diseases that are of public health concern.

A topic of discussion later in the day—the role of organizational structures and independent entities—was introduced at the end of this session. It was noted that a military health professional has other means of reporting problems than strictly to the commander. Outlets outside the chain of command include consultants in the various specialties, inspectors general, and chaplains.

ETHICAL DECISION MAKING: TREATMENT OF DETAINEES

The participants in the second panel discussion considered a case study of ethical challenges to physicians caring for detainees who have undertaken a hunger strike (Box 2). The panel's purpose was to explore

BOX 2

Case Study 2
Treatment of Detainees: Role of Military Health Professionals

Ten detainees in a national security facility have gone on a hunger strike to protest the conditions of their confinement.

Part 1: The strike has gone on for three days, and the detainees are taking only water and vitamins. The camp commander declares the strike a threat to security and order and directs the doctor to evaluate the medical condition of the detainees and to "do whatever is necessary to bring this to an end." The doctor examines the detainees and finds no immediate threat to the health of any individual detainee at this point in the strike.

Part 2: The hunger strike has continued for 45 days. One striker has lost 30 percent of his initial body weight and is felt to be at risk of irreversible harm or even death. He has previously said to the physician that he does not intend to die, but is willing to die if there is no resolution to his grievances.

Considerations:

- What principles are in conflict?
- What guides the clinician in approaching this conflict?
- What about the setting makes this situation different from civilian settings? Are the differences enough to warrant a separate rule? What comparisons are there to civilian settings such as jails and prisons?
- Who is the ultimate decision maker regarding a clinical intervention?
- What mechanisms or resources would help the health professional in resolving this conflict?

broad ethical issues involving treatment of detainees. The context, noted by session moderator Richard J. Bonnie from the University of Virginia, was public concern about treatment of military detainees, including a question of whether physicians have contributed to, or failed to report, certain abuses. The case study, involving a protest against conditions of confinement, included two situations that differed in part in the length of the strike and in directives given to the physician.

International Perspectives

The purpose of a hunger strike—a protest tactic used by Gandhi, by British and American suffragettes, and by Irish Republican Army (IRA) leaders in British prisons—is to shame the authorities. Hernan Reyes, Medical Coordinator for Health in Detention of the International Committee of the Red Cross, stated that hunger strikers do not intend to commit suicide; however, strikers are willing to use their bodies to protest degrading conditions or to promote their cause. To qualify as a hunger strike, a refusal of food must involve "purpose and determination," that is, a willingness to harm oneself if necessary, but only as a *last resort*; the objective is to convince the authorities to respond to the hunger striker's complaints. Reyes differentiated a "food refuser," who does not intend to harm him or herself, from a hunger striker. He also talked about the range in the types of liquids and vitamins taken by hunger strikers. The experience, drawn mostly from the 1981 IRA incident, is that a hunger strike manifests itself within 72 hours, when ketosis[4] can be smelled on the breath, and that death, in those ingesting only water, generally occurs roughly between 55 and 65 days and within a maximum of 73 days.[5]

International declarations support the right of detainees to engage in a hunger strike. The Tokyo Declaration of 1975[6] prohibits artificial feed-

---

[4]*Ketosis* is a metabolic state, associated with starvation, in which the liver excessively converts fat into fatty acids and ketone bodies to use as energy.

[5]The length of survival may depend in part on the prisoner's underlying nutritional status.

[6]"Where a prisoner refuses nourishment and is considered by the physician as capable of forming an unimpaired and rational judgment concerning the consequences of such a voluntary refusal of nourishment, he or she shall not be fed artificially. The decision as to the capacity of the prisoner to form such a judgment should be confirmed by at least one other independent physician. The consequences of the refusal of nourishment shall be explained by the physician to the prisoner" (WMA, 1975).

ing of hunger strikers. Physicians are not supposed to treat hunger strikers so as to send them back to torture. In 2006 the World Medical Association (WMA), with the support of the American Medical Association (AMA), issued the Malta Declaration, stating that physicians are obliged to respect hunger strikers' autonomy (WMA, 2006). The Malta Declaration prohibits force-feeding. It permits artificial feeding, such as the intravenous administration of a saline solution, or even nasogastric feeding, if and only if it is accepted by the hunger striker (WMA, 2006).

Regarding the case study, Reyes noted that a hunger strike of only three days would not require medical intervention. If the strike continues, the physician caring for the hunger striker should consider whether there are specific contraindications, such as diabetes or gastritis, that could lead to permanent adverse effects, even in the case of only a brief strike, and whether the detainee is being coerced into striking through peer pressure from other detainees. The physician should strive to gain the detainee's trust rather than act as an agent of security forces. In the second part of the case, after 45 days, patients would have, or would soon have, ocular-motor problems, including dizziness, inability to stand, and severe vomiting. Most hunger strikers stop fasting when they approach this stage, as it is extremely distressing and uncomfortable. According to the Malta Declaration, consideration is to be given to any advance instructions and patient autonomy respected.

Military Policy

The Department of Defense has adopted a series of policies that govern treatment of hunger strikers. Jack Smith, Director of Clinical and Program Policy Integration in the Office of the Assistant Secretary of Defense for Health Affairs, discussed the principles delineated in 2006 in DoD Instruction 2310.08E (DOD, 2006b):

- Health care personnel have a duty in all matters affecting the physical and mental health of detainees to uphold humane treatment and ensure that detainees are not subject to cruel, inhuman, or degrading treatment or punishment.
- Health care personnel shall not have any provider–patient relationship with detainees "the purpose of which is not solely to evaluate, protect, or improve their physical and mental health."

- Health care personnel charged with the medical care of detainees have a duty to "protect detainees' physical and mental health and provide appropriate treatment for disease"; to the extent feasible, this care should be similar to care provided to U.S. military servicemembers.
- Health care personnel shall not certify or participate in the certification of fitness of detainees for "any form of treatment or punishment that is not in accordance with applicable law, or participate in any way in the administration of any such treatment or punishment."
- Health care personnel are not to participate in application of physical restraints unless such a procedure is "necessary for the protection of the physical or mental health or the safety of the detainee, or necessary for the protection of other detainees or those treating, guarding, or otherwise interacting with them." Health care personnel are not to participate in the custodial physical restraint of detainees.
- Health care is generally provided with consent of the detainee. Detainees have the right to refuse treatment, except for "lifesaving emergency medical care provided to a patient incapable of providing consent or for care necessary to protect public health, such as to prevent the spread of communicable diseases."
- Medical treatment or intervention may be directed without consent of the detainee "in the case of a hunger strike, attempted suicide, or other attempted serious self-harm" when treatment is necessary "to prevent death or serious harm."
- Involuntary treatment must be preceded by a thorough medical and mental health evaluation and counseling concerning the risks and "carried out in a medically appropriate manner." This policy includes "parity," in which detainees are entitled to treatment similar to that provided to U.S. servicemembers.

A decision to undertake compulsory intervention to treat a hunger striker would be made by the joint task force commander, based on the physician's medical assessment and recommendation that "immediate treatment or intervention is necessary to prevent death or serious harm." The procedures are consistent with Federal Bureau of Prisons regulations under Title 28 of the U.S. Code, said Smith, and are designed to support the preservation of life and health by appropriate humane and compassionate clinical intervention when medically necessary.

Regarding the case study, Smith noted that after three days of fasting by a detainee, the physician would conduct a thorough history and physical and mental assessment, and no medical intervention would occur at that point if the patient were found to be healthy. He noted that the first part of the case study was unlikely to occur, because a commander familiar with DoD policy regarding hunger strikers would seek to intervene only when the detainee's life or health was at risk and because commanders typically would call for medical consultations and appropriate specialty referrals. After 45 days of a hunger strike, ethical obligations of beneficence and nonmaleficence would compete with obligations to respect autonomy. Smith questioned whether any confined individual has sufficient autonomy to make a life-or-death decision; hunger strikers could be coerced or acting out of despair or depression.[7]

Smith also noted that under DoD policy, military health professionals are obligated to report suspected or observed abuse to the operational chain of command or, if they do not believe appropriate investigations or actions are occurring, to go through the medical chain of command, the DoD or service inspectors general, or the Criminal Investigative Services.

Correctional Facility Parallels

Scott A. Allen, Co-Director of the Brown University Center for Prison Health and Human Rights, discussed the similarities and differences between the health professional's responsibilities regarding hunger strikers in civilian correctional and military detention environments. Foremost in both settings is the importance of establishing trust with the patient. In the eyes of a patient in either setting, the physician can be perceived as the instrument of the institution. Dual loyalty is an inherent problem in prison medicine and detention facilities, but Allen stressed that the "recognizing of these competing loyalties is not the same as equating them. . . . [L]oyalty to the patient does take preeminence." Similarities also exist in reduced patient autonomy and the physician's limited ability to control events.

---

[7]During the discussion, it was stated that any person refusing food because of coercion or clinical depression is not engaging in a genuine protest fast and that appropriate medical intervention would be permissible to protect the person's health and well-being.

Allen described the potential for a downward spiral of impaired trust in correctional situations that he believes also applies to the military detention situation (Figure 1). The threat of coerced treatment imperils doctor–patient trust, which decreases the chance of resolution, puts pressures on the chain of command to resolve the conflict, and compromises the autonomy of the physician.

Human Rights Perspectives

Although the classic dilemma in the medical response to hunger strikes is a clash between the moral principles of autonomy and beneficence, Leonard S. Rubenstein, President of Physicians for Human Rights, stated that the correct moral decision is clear in cases where human rights violations are occurring. Rubenstein noted that the physician's duty to exercise independent clinical judgment is "woven into the fabric of medical professionalism" and that any command directives seeking to trump those clinical judgments would breach professional standards as well as human rights and the requirements of the Geneva Conventions. Even in a harder case, where a clinical judgment is not dictated but the physician is asked to elevate security interests over the interests of the detainees, Rubenstein stated that the International Dual

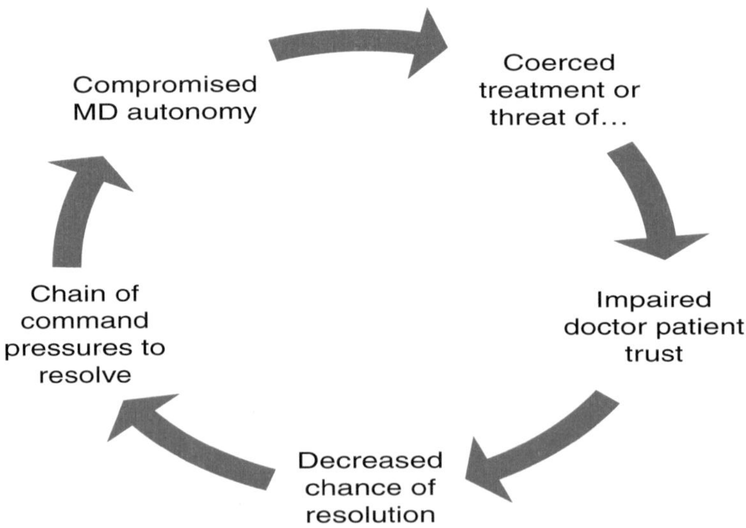

FIGURE 1 Potential for a spiral of impaired trust in prisons.

Loyalty Working Group recommended that any exceptions to patient loyalty by health professionals should be established by competent standard-setting authorities (International Dual Loyalty Working Group, 2003).

In discussing the case study, Rubenstein expanded the hypothetical situations posed by the workshop to include conditions of abuse and other human rights violations against detainees. In such cases the physicians have a duty not merely to *report* abuses, but to try to *stop* the abuses. This requires shaping an environment where physicians are empowered to act ethically, rather than having to resort, in isolation, to heroic tactics to meet their ethical obligations. Most fundamentally, when detainees' human rights are violated, Rubenstein stated that physicians should not use their skills and knowledge to "enable, advance, or permit torture or cruel, inhuman, or degrading maltreatment."

Cultural and Religious Issues

Mahmud A. Thamer, retired Assistant Professor at the Johns Hopkins University School of Medicine and former member of the faculty of Medicine at Baghdad Medical School, asked several leading Islamic scholars of the Sunni and Shi'a traditions about hunger strikes. Asked to define physicians' responsibilities during a hunger strike, the scholars in both sects agreed that a Muslim has no right to undertake a hunger strike that could lead to death unless he or she is prohibited from the performance of religious duties. They also agreed that if the detainees are allowed to practice their religion, it is the responsibility of the attending physician to advise and then actively intervene to stop the hunger strike.

Thamer said it is important to broaden the focus beyond Western individualism and self-determination in order to include cultural viewpoints that emphasize communities, such as those in the Middle East, which have a more tribal and communal perspective. Acknowledging that there are universal human rights, Thamer noted that the manifestations of those rights differ from culture to culture. Similarly, views of what constitutes torture may differ between the West and other cultures; in Islamic societies, for example, sexual humiliation (as practiced to a degree at Abu Ghraib prison in Iraq) is worse than physical blows.

Detention authorities need to consider detainees' cultural traditions and beliefs, Thamer said. Authorities could involve religious and tribal leaders in creating an atmosphere of respect and order that can increase compliance.

Discussion

Reyes began the discussion session by emphasizing that the clinician should consider the specific circumstances of each case before taking a course of action, offering as an illustration a recent case in which a judge and a physician disagreed about whether to force-feed a self-styled hunger striker who at the three-week point of the strike was not at clinical risk and who was being manipulative. In addition to determining whether there are indications of depression or other mental illnesses, health professionals should consult individually with each hunger striker to determine whether he or she has been subjected to peer pressure or coercion.

The participants discussed the differences between the DoD policy and the WMA Malta Declaration. During the discussion it was noted that permitting forcible treatment of mentally competent hunger strikers contravenes the WMA 2006 Malta Declaration and the official position of the American Medical Association. Further, it was noted that a command decision overriding the medical recommendation, although unlikely to occur, would also violate the Malta Declaration. Smith stated that the DoD policy's emphasis on beneficence and preservation of life can create trust on the part of detainees toward medical professionals, who will act to prevent medical harm if possible. Furthermore, Smith noted, the policy prevents radical leaders from imposing a hunger strike on less powerful prisoners. A workshop participant suggested that the different positions of the DoD and WMA should be brought to a neutral authoritative body, such as state boards that license U.S. civilian and military physicians.

One participant stated that he felt that there was agreement of the participants that commanders should not overrule the professional medical judgment of physicians. However, there were differences of opinion among participants about the actual conditions of confinement and interrogation previously in place at Guantanamo (and about the extent to which these conditions have since been ameliorated). Several participants pushed for further inquiries into allegations of past abuse.

Allen commented, from personal experience, about the risks that whistle-blowers encounter. Several participants emphasized the importance of ensuring multiple avenues for reporting ethical concerns and not relying on medical heroism. Along these lines, DoD representatives discussed the multiple avenues that are available to health professionals in detainee facilities including both the line and medical chains of command, medical specialty consultants, law enforcement officials, and service or DoD inspectors general. Participants also stressed the need to ensure the viability and accessibility of these options, as well as the need to broadly disseminate this information.

The value of transparency was highlighted by several participants as was the need to achieve the highest possible level of transparency consistent with national security. Also acknowledged were positive changes that have been made at Guantanamo and the professionalism of many military health professionals. Productive efforts to engage both human rights organizations and military health professionals in discussions about the revisions to the Army field manual on interrogation were highlighted.

Several matters were also raised for further consideration. Bruce Meneley, commander of the Joint Medical Group at Guantanamo, asked about a physician's ethical obligation toward people who use martyrdom as a tactic. Panel moderator Richard Bonnie raised the issue of the physician's role as a mediator or negotiator, which complicates the already numerous roles of the health care professional in conducting assessments of the hunger striker's health status, capacity, and motivation, as well as providing counseling. Mediating between the patient and the commander, while remaining loyal to both sides, is difficult at best. Another participant supported greater consideration of cultural aspects by policy makers.

INITIAL AFTERNOON DISCUSSION

The afternoon session opened with a general discussion of the morning's presentations. Planning Committee Chair Childress asked how to delineate when a health professional is in the role of health care provider and is therefore in a provider–patient relationship: Is this defined by the nature of the relationship (such as a person being brought to the physician for an examination) or by the use of the physician's knowledge and skills (such as the physician's perception of an absence of proper care)? Linda Emanuel raised an additional question: When should someone (such as an on-base fellow officer of a psychiatrist) be regarded as a potential patient to whom the physician may owe a duty of confidentiality and other safeguards? Further, at what point should a health professional be advocating for a solution to the root cause of the problem?

One participant responded that in hospitals or other institutional settings, the physician assumes a duty to the patient early on as an agent of an institution that is clearly responsible for caring for the patient. For example, as soon as an injured individual comes into the emergency room, health care professionals initiate the provider–patient relationship. In other cases, the patient's perception of the fiduciary relationship may be a factor in determining the physician's scope of duty. Addressing the operational military context, another participant said that because the commander makes the ultimate decision and may need to place the mission's interest above the individual's interest, the physician should represent the patient. It was also noted that a presumption of confidentiality exists in the military, with some stated exceptions, so a physician–patient relationship exists even in the case of prisoners.

Discussion also turned to the many challenges that arise in operational settings such as Iraq, where health professionals may be caring for a range of patients—U.S. and allied troops, U.S. and allied civilians, Iraqi civilians, and enemy combatants—and may need to make decisions about priority of care while also taking into account security concerns.

ETHICS TRAINING

The participants in the third panel discussion considered approaches to informing or instructing physicians (and other military health professionals and health care workers) about ethical issues.

Training of Military Medical Students

According to recent empirical evidence, most U.S. medical students and military physicians are generally uninformed about medical ethical issues in military medicine (Bloche and Marks, 2005; Boyd et al., 2007). To remedy these deficiencies, Edmund Howe, Professor of Psychiatry at the Uniformed Services University of the Health Sciences (USUHS), stressed the importance of teaching ethics to future military physicians. In part because of dual loyalties, the military setting can present ethical situations that differ from typical civilian situations. For example, military triage decisions in time of battle—such as the classic example from

World War II of who should first receive antibiotics that are in short supply—reflect the utilitarian goal of the greatest good for the greatest number, rather than a standard of treating the sickest patients first.

Howe noted three ethical precepts that are centrally applicable to treatment of prisoners and that are just as relevant to situations in military medicine:

- equality or parity in treating patients,
- elasticity or flexibility in implementing policies, and
- the historic principle of "first, do no harm" (*primum non nocere*).

Precisely because of their dual roles as agents of the military and clinicians, military physicians should clarify any ambiguities for the patient, who may not always perceive which hat the physician is wearing. For example, when taking a medical history and asking about substance abuse, the physician should tell the patient up-front about the health professional's obligations if illegal drug use is reported.

In teaching ethics at USUHS, Howe and colleagues use several approaches. Invited speakers who can share their ethical dilemmas through classroom presentations and discussions serve as models of appropriate decision making. Other approaches include case study discussions and field practice exercises in which superior officers issue simulated orders, some of which may be unethical, and students are asked to decide how to proceed. Students also learn about the different chains of command and to whom they can report activities that they suspect may be unethical.

Ethics Training in the Field and Continuing Education

Ethics training can also take place through opportunities for continuing education. Kenneth W. Schor, Assistant Professor of Preventive Medicine and Biometrics at USUHS, described an ethics training course that was implemented with personnel on the hospital ship *USNS Mercy* as it traveled the South Pacific as part of Pacific Partnership 2008. The ethics course was accredited for both continuing medical education and continuing nursing education. Participants included not only military health professionals but also U.S. Public Health Service staff of the Commissioned Corps, civilian volunteers from organizations such as Project HOPE and Operation Smile, and personnel from partner nations.

The instruction occurred during transits between ports, as those were the teachable moments when personnel were on board and no one was actively treating patients. In providing care quickly overseas to thousands of victims of natural disasters or epidemics, these health care workers and volunteers must balance the health of individual patients with the health of the population. The ethics course was case-based and included structured discussion; this format elicited a great deal of discussion about personal experiences. The training also adapted a human rights impact assessment tool for public health interventions and policies (Box 3). Schor noted the dearth of peer-reviewed literature on the ethics of humanitarian assistance as well as the need for ethical considerations to "seep" into the planning, implementation, and assessment phases of humanitarian assistance missions.

BOX 3

Adapted Human Rights Impact Assessment Tool for Public Health Interventions and Policies

1. Is there a clearly defined compelling and justified public health purpose?
2. Is the program/policy appropriate and likely to be efficient and effective?
3. Is the intervention well-targeted (neither overly inclusive nor under-inclusive)?
4. Are any civil, political, social, economic, or cultural rights being infringed upon or any ethical principles being violated?
5. Are there alternative interventions that are less intrusive/invasive or that have fewer ethical encumbrances?
6. Is the intervention likely to avert significant harm?
7. Are there procedural safeguards in place to ensure equity, fairness, and accountability?
8. Are the decision-making and intervention processes transparent to all concerned?

SOURCE: Adapted from Gostin and Mann (1994).

Scenarios presented in the onboard training exercises included

- conflict between the opinions of health professionals and force protection rules—for example, when surgical complications arise and overnight care for the patient could compromise the medical team's safety;
- the impact on the host nations—for example, the impact of the mission on the livelihood of local physicians and other health professionals;
- questions about whose standard of care should prevail when U.S. health professionals practice in another country;
- resource allocation decisions and public communication needs when more patients arrive to be treated than can be cared for; and
- the importance of being knowledgeable about and respecting cultural traditions in the host country.

Improving the Teaching of Ethics

Experiences in teaching medical ethics in palliative care and geriatrics—disciplines that concentrate on the whole person rather than on disease processes—could inform training in medical ethics in a range of contexts. Joshua Hauser, Assistant Director of the Northwestern University Buehler Center on Aging, Health & Society, noted that ethical issues in palliative care include medical futility, informed consent, assisted suicide, autonomy, and team responsibility.

Efforts to improve education in palliative care are led by the Education in Palliative and End-of-life Care Project, which has included a focus on ethics education. Students have complained that ethics training can be too abstract or boring. The following are some basic principles found to improve the teaching of ethics to health professionals:

- Make it real—use real patients and real situations.
- Make it novel—challenge the students' assumptions and use new approaches to connect the patient and student.
- Make it engaging.
- Make it convenient.
- Make it relevant.

Hauser has found the greatest success in teaching ethics by engaging students directly in both structured and unstructured situations and applying novel education methods, such as multiprofessional conversations (sometimes termed "Schwartz Center Rounds"[8]), role play, videotaped interviews with patients, and community settings. (For illustrative purposes, he played a videotape excerpt of an interview with a terminally ill lung cancer patient discussing her interactions with comfort caregivers.) Videos allow the instructor to bring out different aspects of the patient's care and specific ethical issues while focusing on the realities of the situation.

Opportunities for ethics training exist throughout the training process. For example, in the first two years of medical school, students can follow patients longitudinally under close faculty supervision. During clinical years, students can interact with patients in different contexts and will encounter broader issues through interactions with family members and others involved in the care of the patient.

Discussion

Howe, who moderated the session, asked whether more patient-centered videos should be produced to serve as a core method of teaching medical ethics and, if so, when they should be shown and to whom. Schor answered that they should be shown at the start of medical missions and commented that in the onboard exercises, participants such as military physicians and Project HOPE volunteers enjoyed learning each other's perspectives. Emerging information technologies offer exciting opportunities for disseminating and sharing information, opinions, and experiences regarding ethical challenges.

Developing ethics training that is real, practical, and timely requires choosing material that relates to the learning objectives. Policy issues can be perceived from the top down, such as who decides, or from the bottom up, such as how to deal with uncertainties. Problems that arise in medical practice often can be identified by asking students to recount an experience when they were not sure of the right action to take. While

[8]Schwartz Center Rounds engage physicians, nurses, social workers, students, and other health professionals in interdisciplinary rounds in the hospital or other health care setting. Named for an attorney in Massachusetts who felt that his professional caregivers needed to improve their communications with each other, the Kenneth B. Schwartz Center funds these efforts around the country (Kenneth B. Schwartz Center, 2008).

preserving the productive and important tension between commanders and military health professionals, continuing education provides a means for discerning the two groups' mutual interests and learning practical ways of realizing them.

INSTILLING ETHICAL VALUES: ORGANIZATIONAL STRUCTURE AND CULTURE

The participants in the fourth panel discussion considered how organizational structure and culture can affect, nurture, and sustain ethical values. Organizations are living systems that have moral capacity and that are accountable to stakeholders for their standards of purpose and value. Session moderator Linda Emanuel, Director of the Northwestern University Buehler Center on Aging, Health & Society, explained that such standards determine an organization's culture, structure, processes, and outcomes. Emanuel said that the present discourse between the medical profession and the military should lead to standards that would apply across sectors and disciplines—which have interdependent and balanced roles—and could evolve through continuous learning.

Nurturing a Just Culture

What is a just organization? David T. Ozar, Professor of Philosophy at Loyola University of Chicago, posited that a just organization affirms the role it assigns to its members to make complex ethics-laden decisions. Further, it supports these decisions by providing necessary communications, education, and other organizational processes. A just organization communicates openly about decisions after the fact to effect improvements, and it commends rather than punishes individuals for bringing ethical issues to light. At all levels, Ozar suggested, a just organization demonstrates adherence to its professed values.

Organizations can influence ethical conduct, according to Ozar, through positive impact on their members' ethical awareness, judgment, motivation, and implementation. A just organization, he said,

- fosters a rich awareness of, and sensibility for, its stated values and ideals, not just in generalities but in ways linked to actual decisions "on the ground," rather than leaving individuals to their own devices, and it tests its structures and processes to ensure that they are producing ethical results;

- emphasizes the complexity of ethical decisions and the difficult judgments they require, provides resources to support individuals' ethical reflection and judgment, and commends individuals for displaying such reflection and judgment (e.g., in the military context, neither commanders in theater nor superiors within the medical hierarchy should expect physicians to act in isolation or blame them for ethical decisions not anticipated by rules and regulations);
- supports the positive motivations of its members by focusing its systems on positive values rather than using coercion and fear to attain results, and responds to ethical lapses first of all as organizational issues rather than personal aberrations; and
- actively assists its members to implement ethics consistently by identifing barriers to ethical conduct, developing a repertoire of interventions to assist individuals in making ethical decisions, and establishing a communication system for promoting ethical decision making before, during, and after an event. In this connection, most lapses in implementation can be attributed either to psychological barriers, such as fear and hopelessness, or practical barriers, in which the individual does not know how to decide or where to turn for consultation.

To illustrate the importance of dialogue about these components of ethical conduct with members of an organization at all levels, Ozar recounted the changes at one hospital that occurred through asking employees about impediments to realizing the hospital's core values. After hearing a patient transport assistant's concern about having to leave patients isolated on gurneys without a way for them to summon assistance, the hospital responded by reconfiguring the units so that waiting patients could see and be seen by a receptionist. Respectful and serious conversations with people on the ground can lead to important systems and organizational changes that can markedly increase the chances that the organization's values and ethical standards will be actualized in its members' judgments and conduct.

Leadership and Vertical Integration

No substitute exists for leadership that is explicitly, materially (through the dedication of resources), and passionately committed to the ethical pursuit of an organization's mission. Daniel D. Federman, Professor of Medicine and Medical Education at Harvard Medical School, said that the commander sets the tone and that, ideally, the highest levels of leadership communicate their commitment to ethics with the same emphasis as other goals. Federman stressed the need to review allegations of ethical infractions quickly and as publicly as possible.

An ombudsperson function was added at Harvard Medical School over 17 years ago to hear and investigate, confidentially, complaints about administrative malfunctions—or, more broadly, any institution-related concerns. An ombudsperson is, in large measure, a listener, with access to many sources of information and the responsibility to report on anonymous complaints. The Harvard ombudsperson issues a broadly disseminated annual report that reveals patterns and trends; in this way, an individual's confidential complaint carries weight as part of aggregated information. For example, frequently expressed complaints have led to improvements, or at least heightened sensitivity, in the areas of sexual harassment, research integrity, and intellectual property at the medical school. Reports are provided by the ombudsperson's office in many settings to get the messages to multiple key audiences in the medical school, including the administration, faculty, new employees, managers, mentors, and the human relations office. The cumulative impact of the *ombuds* function is to hold up a mirror, allowing the institution to reshape itself if it does not like what it sees, said Federman.

Learning and Accountability in Organizational Structures

What are next steps in making organizations more ethically attuned? Emanuel discussed building learning and layered accountability into organizations. Ensuring that organizations act ethically requires layered stages of professional voices, including an external voice, she said, as well as organizational feedback, deliberation, organized advocacy, and disobedience when necessary.

Conflicts of interest provide an example of an ethical problem that can be addressed through a set of approaches appropriate to the level of ethical concern. Under current rules in force in most settings, some conflicts are flatly prohibited, some are limited, and some are merely disclosed, depending on a variety of factors, namely, the sum of money at stake, the proximity of the conflict to patient care, and the values involved. Checks and balances within an organizational structure are not necessarily sufficient to prevent undue conflicts of interest from arising. For example, at the American Medical Association (AMA), accountability appeared to translate well into the structure. However, in 1997 AMA entered into a marketing agreement with the Sunbeam Corporation[9] that violated the organization's ethical principles. In addressing this situation, AMA found that the problem had resulted from a lack of transparency coupled with poor decision making. The challenge after a major lapse is to learn from the mistakes and work to restore positive culture and leadership, Emanuel said.

Structural mechanisms useful for promoting medical ethics within a health care organization include

- peer review;
- advisory boards;
- institutional review boards, for investigative research;
- systems engineering and continuous learning and improvement (in the patient safety area, for example, effective approaches incorporate teamwork and opportunities for speaking against the authority gradient and for both anonymous and compulsory reporting of lapses); and
- involvement of multiple professions, such as clergy, educators, and social workers.

As the military continues in its efforts as a learning organization, it is important to identify, refine, and institutionalize mechanisms for continued deliberation on issues in military medical ethics.

Discussion

The panel members had an opportunity for discussion followed by general discussion with the workshop participants. One barrier to organization-wide ethical behavior is the "myth of enough good people," Ozar

[9]The marketing agreement allowed Sunbeam to display the AMA logo on packages of its products, regardless of whether the product provided a demonstrated health benefit.

remarked. According to this myth, if we just recruit enough good people—the best and the brightest—into our organization, we will not have any ethical problems.

Lieutenant General Eric Schoomaker, U.S. Army Surgeon General, commented that the discussion in the workshop had recognized that the ethical issues faced by military health professionals are a microcosm of ethical issues faced by the larger medical community in the United States. Some ethical conflicts arise from situations in which there is a misunderstanding about servicemember's rights, such as the right of the individual, under ordinary circumstances, to refuse treatment. Further efforts are needed to continue to examine competing ethical principles and to explore the concerns about security to ensure the highest level of transparency that is feasible.

Several participants noted that there are a number of organizational structures in place in the military that support whistle-blowing, including ombudsperson offices and ethics experts who are outside the normal chain of command. Although these structures appear to be transparent and known by military health professionals, they are apparently less familiar to their civilian counterparts.

CONCLUSIONS AND NEXT STEPS

The workshop concluded with James Childress summarizing the day's discussions, Joseph Kelley providing his thoughts on next steps, and workshop participants presenting final thoughts.

Childress summarized the presentations and discussions during the workshop in the following 10 points:

1. The need for transparency in policies and processes related to military ethics was affirmed, as were the challenges in further achieving it both internally and externally.
2. Military medical ethics discussions benefit from a wide range of public and professional perspectives.
3. In addressing medical ethics issues, we need to attend—imaginatively and thoughtfully—to diverse social and cultural views, beliefs, and practices.
4. Organizational structures, systems, training, and procedures need to be in place so that individual actors do not have to act heroically to ensure ethically proper decisions.

5. International and domestic laws supporting medical ethics are essential but do not obviate the need for ethical analysis.
6. Codes of ethics help to guide ethical behavior by physicians and other health professionals but are not specific enough to address each individual ethical issue that comes up in clinical practice.
7. Similarities and differences between dual loyalties in the military and dual loyalties in other fields, such as occupational and sports medicine, are illuminating and instructive.
8. Patient trust in health care professionals is vital, yet difficult to engender in circumstances of dual loyalty.
9. Ethical dilemmas can be either *intra-agent*—reflecting situations when different moral principles conflict—or *inter-agent,* such as between a military commander and a physician.
10. Ethical decision making requires more than prioritizing separate principles, such as autonomy and beneficence. The principles must be made concrete and ways found to be as specific as possible about how to apply them in practice.

Childress emphasized this last point by stating that ethical principles alone may not provide enough practical guidance. Ongoing efforts focused on defining specific ethical responsibilities are needed in certain settings.

Kelley began his summary of the workshop by highlighting the concept of the triad—patient, physician, commander—and emphasizing the need for communication. Although the workshop focused primarily on the policy perspective, it will be important for future discussions, Kelley noted, to focus on the perspective of the practitioner. Kelley stressed that the military is not monolithic but has provisions in place for military health professionals to exercise their right of conscience, including support for health professionals who have ethical concerns and are seeking to determine ethical courses of action. This right applies to physicians who are dealing with situations such as hunger strikes. He noted, too, that the organization is what makes the individual effective while realizing that national security concerns must be addressed. Opportunities for ethics training can draw from the models presented in the workshop.

Kelley emphasized the need for as much transparency as possible. He encouraged allegations of situations of concern to be shared with available information so that they can be investigated. Further, he emphasized the need for continued dialogue on ethical issues between the military and civilian medical communities.

In the discussion that followed, participants raised several points, including

- The hunger strike case study demonstrates the need for further development of ethical guidelines for military health professionals as well as further discussions to more fully understand the nature of ethical concerns and the extent of opportunities for professional autonomy by military health professionals.
- The military is not monolithic, and military physicians have substantial professional autonomy, so similar dilemmas can produce different results.
- Further discussions are needed on the structures or systems that the military has (or could have) in place to assist not only physicians but also other health professionals, such as psychologists, in situations where they are serving as behavioral science consultants.
- The military has provided greatly increased guidance on medical ethics since 2006, including a substantial body of policy and standard operating procedures at the operational level. The DoD continues to be a learning organization on issues raised by detainee treatment—including hunger strikes, forensic roles, and training—and dual loyalty.
- Increased attention to ensuring the transparency of DoD policy, guidelines, and protocols is an ongoing need with the understanding that national security issues will be addressed. There is strong interest in continuing to find common ground and in discussing ethical issues integral to hunger strike management, interrogation policies, and other related issues.

Discussion also focused on additional next steps for open dialogue, including the formation of advisory committees to DoD through either the National Academies or other entities. These types of committees can review events involving challenging ethical components and recommend policy improvements, a mechanism that has been used by other national security–related agencies. Recent and ongoing changes in the Defense Health Board in this direction were noted, and appreciation was expressed for the opportunity in this workshop to have open and reasoned dialogue with individuals with a wide range of expertise and interest. Several participants noted that interrogation issues have been controversial, and it was suggested that a forum specifically exploring these issues might be useful.

A

References

ACOEM (American College of Occupational and Environmental Medicine). 2008. ACOEM code of ethical conduct. http://www.acoem.org/codeofconduct.aspx (accessed 10/22/2008).

Beam, T. E., and L. R. Sparacino. 2003. Military Medical Ethics. Washington, DC: Borden Institute. Volumes 1 and 2. http://www.bordeninstitute.army.mil/published.html (accessed 10/22/2008).

Bloche, M. G., and J. H. Marks. 2005. When doctors go to war. New England Journal of Medicine 352(1):3–6.

Boyd, J. W., D. U. Himmelstein, K. Lasser, D. McCormick, D. H. Bor, S. L. Cutrona, and S. Woolhandler. 2007. U.S. medical students' knowledge about the military draft, the Geneva Conventions, and military medical ethics. International Journal of Health Services 37(4):643–650.

DoD (U.S. Department of Defense). 2006a. Policy guidance for deployment-limiting psychiatric conditions and medications. http://www.health.mil/Content/docs/pdfs/policies/2006/Guidance_20061107_deplo_limiting_psyc_cond.pdf (accessed 10/30/2008).

DoD. 2006b. Instruction: Medical program support for detainee operations. Number2310.08E. http://www.js.pentagon.mil/whs/directives/corres/pdf/231008p.pdf (accessed 10/22/2008).

Gostin, L., and J. M. Mann. 1994. Towards the development of a human rights impact assessment for the formulation and evaluation of public health policies. Health and Human Rights 1(1):58–80.

ICOH (International Commission on Occupational Health). 2002. International code of ethics for occupational health professionals. http://www.icohweb.org/core_docs/code_ethics_eng.pdf (accessed 10/22/2008).

International Dual Loyalty Working Group. 2003. Dual loyalty and human rights in health professional practice: Proposed guidelines and institutional mechanisms. Cambridge, MA: Physicians for Human Rights.

Johnson, W. B., R. Bacho, M. Heim, and J. Ralph. 2006. Multiple-role dilemmas for military mental health care providers. Military Medicine 171(4): 311–315.

Kenneth B. Schwartz Center. 2008. Schwartz Center Rounds. http://www.theschwartzcenter.org/programs/rounds.html (accessed 10/22/2008).

Strasburger, L. H., T. G. Gutheil, and A. Brodsky. 1997. On wearing two hats: Role conflict in serving as both psychotherapist and expert witness. American Journal of Psychiatry 154(4):448–456.

U.S. Army. 2004. Oaths of enlistment and oaths of office. http://www.history.army.mil/faq/oaths.htm (accessed 10/22/2008).

WMA (World Medical Association). 1975. Declaration of Tokyo. Guideline for physicians concerning torture and other cruel, inhuman or degrading treatment or punishment in relation to detention and imprisonment. Adopted by the 29th World Medical Assembly, Tokyo, Japan, October 1975, and editorially revised in May 2005 and May 2006, Divonne-les-Bains, France. http://www.wma.net/e/policy/c18.htm (accessed 10/22/2008).

WMA. 2006. Declaration on hunger strikers. Adopted by the 43rd World Medical Assembly, Malta, November 1991, and editorially revised at the 44th World Medical Assembly, Marbella, Spain, September 1992, and revised by the WMA General Assembly, Pilanesberg, South Africa, October 2006. http://www.wma.net/e/policy/h31.htm (accessed 10/22/2008).

B

Workshop Agenda

INSTITUTE OF MEDICINE
National Academy of Sciences

Workshop on Military Medical Ethics:
Issues Regarding Dual Loyalties

Monday, September 8, 2008
National Academy of Sciences
Lecture Room
2100 C Street, NW
Washington, DC

Workshop Goals

- Examine ethical challenges for physicians and other health professionals serving in the military that arise from conflicts between their responsibilities to patients and their duties as military officers
- Discuss parallels with other fields of health and draw on their efforts to develop ethical guidelines and training models
- Discuss effective organizational structures that support and promote a just work culture

7:30 a.m. **Continental Breakfast**

8:00 **Welcome and Opening Remarks**
James Childress, Chair
Harvey Fineberg, President, Institute of Medicine
Joseph Kelley, Deputy Assistant Secretary of Defense for Clinical and Program Policy

8:40 **Setting the Context for the Discussion**
James Childress, Chair

9:00 **Case Study 1: Return to Duty: Ethical Issues for Military Health Professionals**
Moderator: Paul Appelbaum, Columbia University

9:00–10:00 Panel Presentations

- Outline of the Case and Issues
  Paul Appelbaum, Columbia University
- Military Policy and Data
  Elspeth Cameron Ritchie, U.S. Army
- Parallels in Occupational Health
  Myron Harrison, ExxonMobil
- Parallels in Sports Medicine
  Kurt Spindler, Vanderbilt University

10:00–10:30 Panel Discussion

10:30–10:45 General Discussion

10:45 **Break**

11:00 **Case Study 2: Treatment of Detainees: Role of Military Health Professionals**
Moderator: Richard Bonnie, University of Virginia

11:00–12:15 Panel Presentations

- Introduction and Outline of the Case
  Richard Bonnie, University of Virginia

- Overview of the Issues
  Hernan Reyes, International Committee of the Red Cross
- Military Policy
  Jack Smith, Department of Defense
- Parallels in Correctional and Custodial Facilities
  Scott Allen, Brown University
- Human Rights Issues
  Leonard Rubenstein, Physicians for Human Rights
- Intercultural and Religious Issues
  Mahmud Thamer, Johns Hopkins University

12:15–12:45 Panel Discussion

12:45–1:00 General Discussion

1:00 p.m. **Lunch**

1:45 **General Discussion—Follow-up from Morning Discussions**
Moderator: James Childress

2:15 **Ethics Training for Military Health Professionals**
Moderator: Randy Howe, Uniformed Services University of the Health Sciences (USUHS)

2:15–2:55 Panel Presentations

- Ethics Training at the Uniformed Services University of the Health Sciences
  Randy Howe, USUHS
- Ethics Training in the Field and Continuing Education
  Kenneth Schor, USUHS
- Improving the Teaching of Ethics
  Joshua Hauser, Northwestern University

2:55–3:15 Panel and General Discussion

3:15 **Ethical Values—Organizational Structure and Culture**

Moderator: Linda Emanuel, Northwestern University

3:15–3:50 Panel Presentations

- Overview of the Issues
  Linda Emanuel, Northwestern University
- Nurturing a Just Culture
  David Ozar, Loyola University, Chicago
- Leadership and Vertical Integration
  Daniel Federman, Harvard University
- Learning and Accountability Within Organizational Structures: Where Next?
  Linda Emanuel, Northwestern University

3:50–4:15 Panel and General Discussion

4:15 Next Steps

James Childress, Chair
Joseph Kelley, Deputy Assistant Secretary of Defense for Clinical and Program Policy

5:00 Adjourn

C

Workshop Participants List

Peter Agre
University Professor and Director
Johns Hopkins Malaria Research Institute

Scott A. Allen
Co-Director, Center for Prisoner Health and Human Rights
Alpert Medical School
Brown University

George Annas
Professor and Chair
Boston University School of Public Health

Paul S. Appelbaum
Elizabeth K. Dollard Professor of Psychiatry, Medicine, and Law
Columbia University Medical Center, New York Psychiatric Institute

Louie Banks
U.S. Army

Thomas E. Beam
COL (retired), MC, U.S. Army

Bill Blazek
Assistant Professor of Medicine
Research Scholar
Center for Clinical Bioethics
Georgetown University School of Medicine

David Blazes
Head
Global Emerging Infections System
Armed Forces Health Surveillance Center

Richard J. Bonnie
Harrison Foundation Professor of Medicine and Law
Professor of Psychiatry and Neurobehavioral Sciences
Director, Institute of Law, Psychiatry, and Public Policy
University of Virginia

John Bradshaw
Washington Director
Physicians for Human Rights

Franklin Branch
Research Associate
Board on Health Sciences Policy
Institute of Medicine

Nori Y. Buising
Medical Corps
Deputy Director, Medical Education
Office of the Surgeon General

James F. Childress
John Allen Hollingsworth Professor of Ethics
Director, Institute for Practical Ethics and Public Life
University of Virginia

Sarah Comley
International Observer

Paul Cordts
Director, Health Policy and Services
Office of the Surgeon General

Carol Corillon
Director, Committee on Human Rights
National Academies

Soo Lee Davis
Office of the Surgeon General

Chaplain David Deppmeier
Clinical Ethicist
Walter Reed Army Medical Center

William Dunn
U.S. Air Force

Linda Emanuel
Buehler Professor of Geriatric Medicine
Director, Buehler Center on Aging, Health & Society
Northwestern University

Ellen Embrey
Deputy Assistant Secretary of Defense for Force Health Protection and Readiness

Marcus Eng
Experient, Inc.

Rick Erdtmann
Director, Board on Military and Veterans Health and the Medical Follow-up Agency
Institute of Medicine

Judy Estep
Program Associate
Board on Health Sciences Policy
Institute of Medicine

Daniel D. Federman
Carl W. Walter Distinguished Professor of Medicine and Medical Education
Harvard Medical School

Harvey Fineberg
President
Institute of Medicine

Edward Gabriele
Special Assistant for Ethics & Professional Integrity
USN Bureau of Medicine and Surgery
Office of the Surgeon General of the Navy

Bruce Green
Air Force Deputy Surgeon General
Office of the Air Force Surgeon General

Sara Greenberg
Physicians for Human Rights

Amy Haas
Administrative Assistant
Board on Health Sciences Policy
Institute of Medicine

Myron C. Harrison
Senior Health Adviser
ExxonMobil Corporation

Joshua Hauser
Assistant Director
Buehler Center on Aging, Health & Society
Palliative Care and Home Hospice Program
Feinberg School of Medicine
Northwestern University

Edmund Howe
Professor of Psychiatry
Uniformed Services University of the Health Sciences

Sandral Hullett
CEO and Medical Director
Cooper Green Hospital

Jeffrey Janofsky
Associate Professor
Johns Hopkins University

Thomas C. Jefferson
Consultant, Ethics, to Army Surgeon General
U.S. Army

Tyrone Jefferson
Industrial and Organizational Psychologist
Aptima Inc.

Jason Kaar
Uniformed Services University of the Health Sciences

Joseph Kelley
Deputy Assistant Secretary of Defense for Clinical and Program Policy
Department of Defense

Linda Kilroy
Contract Manager
Office of Contracts and Grants
National Academy of Sciences

Catharyn T. Liverman
Project Director
Board on Health Sciences Policy
Institute of Medicine

Bruce Meneley
Joint Medical Group, Joint Task Force, Guantanamo
U.S. Naval Hospital

Timothy Murphy
Professor of Philosophy in the Biomedical Sciences
University of Illinois College of Medicine

Elena Nightingale
Scholar-in-Residence
Institute of Medicine

Susan Okie
National Correspondent
New England Journal of Medicine

David T. Ozar
Professor
Philosophy Department
Loyola University, Chicago

Jennifer Peters
Dewitt Army Community Hospital

Ellen Pinholt
Walter Reed Army Medical Center

Andrew M. Pope
Director
Board on Health Sciences Policy
Institute of Medicine

Joseph Procaccino
Legal Adviser to the Surgeon General
U.S. Air Force

Hernan Reyes
Medical Coordinator
Health in Detention
International Committee of the Red Cross

Elspeth Cameron Ritchie
Medical Director, Strategic Communication
Army Medical Department

M. E. Bonnie Rogers
Associate Professor of Nursing and Public Health
University of North Carolina School of Public Health

Leonard S. Rubenstein
President
Physicians for Human Rights

Eric Schoomaker
Army Surgeon General
Office of the Surgeon General
U.S. Army

Kenneth W. Schor
Assistant Professor
Preventive Medicine and Biometrics
Uniformed Services University of the Health Sciences

Adil Shamoo
Professor
Department of Biochemistry and Molecular Biology
University of Maryland Baltimore

David Smith
Joint Staff Surgeon
The Joint Staff

Jack Smith
Director, Clinical and Program Policy Integration
Office of the Assistant Secretary of Defense for Health Affairs

Ronald Sollock
Bureau of Medicine and Surgery

Mildred Z. Solomon
Associate Professor of Social Medicine and Medical Ethics
Harvard Medical School

Kurt P. Spindler
Professor, Orthopaedics and Rehabilitation
Vanderbilt University School of Medicine

William Stubing
President
The Greenwall Foundation

Kathleen Sullivan
Chief Program Officer
Physicians for Human Rights

Mahmud A. Thamer
Assistant Professor of Medicine, (retired)
Johns Hopkins University

Gerald Thomson
Professor of Medicine Emeritus
Columbia University

Neil Weisfeld
Principal
New Associates, LLC

Vicki Weisfeld
Principal
New Associates, LLC

Stephen N. Xenakis
Physicians for Human Rights

Howard Zonana
Director, Yale Law and Psychiatry Division
Yale University School of Medicine

D

Biographical Sketches of Workshop Speakers and Planning Committee Members

WORKSHOP SPEAKERS

Daniel D. Federman, M.D., is the Senior Dean of Clinical Teaching at Harvard Medical School. An endocrinologist by training, Dr. Federman maintains active clinical practices at Brigham and Women's Hospital and Harvard University Health Services. Dr. Federman served on the faculty of Harvard Medical School from 1960 to 1972 and was simultaneously on the staff of Massachusetts General Hospital. From 1972 to 1977 he was chairman of the Department of Medicine at Stanford Medical School. He then returned to Harvard Medical School as Dean for Students and Alumni and Professor of Medicine. In 1989 he was appointed Dean for Medical Education and in 1992 was named the Carl W. Walter Professor of Medicine and Medical Education. Dr. Federman has served as Chairman of the American Board of Internal Medicine and President of the American College of Physicians and is a member of the Institute of Medicine. He was one of the founding editors of Scientific American® Medicine. Dr. Federman has received from the American College of Physicians both the Massachusetts Physician of the Year and the Distinguished Teacher awards, as well as The Endocrine Society's Distinguished Educator Award. In 2001 the Association of American Medical Colleges honored him with their Abraham Flexner Award for Distinguished Service to Medical Education. Born in New York City, Dr. Federman received his A.B. from Harvard College and his M.D. from Harvard Medical School.

Harvey V. Fineberg, M.D., Ph.D., is President of the Institute of Medicine. He previously served Harvard University as Provost and as Dean of the School of Public Health. Dr. Fineberg also has served as President of the Society for Medical Decision Making and consultant to the World Health Organization. His research has included assessment of medical technology, evaluation of vaccines, and dissemination of medical innovations. He is the author or coauthor of numerous books and articles on subjects ranging from AIDS prevention to medical education. Dr. Fineberg holds four degrees from Harvard, including an M.D. and a Ph.D. in public policy.

Myron Harrison, M.D., M.P.H., is the Senior Health Adviser for ExxonMobil and a member of its corporate Safety, Health and Environment staff. Previously he served as the Medical Director of Exxon's U.S. Medicine and Occupational Health Department. Before specializing in the field of occupational medicine, he practiced emergency medicine for 10 years. Dr. Harrison earned a master of public health degree at Columbia University and is a Past President of the Texas College of Occupational and Environmental Medicine. He is an Adjunct Professor at the University of Texas School of Public Health, where he teaches "Ethical Dilemmas in Occupational Medicine."

Joshua M. Hauser, M.D., is an Assistant Professor in Medicine and Palliative Care; Director of the Education Section and Assistant Director of the Buehler Center on Aging, Health & Society; and Director of the Education in Palliative and End-of-life Care Project at Northwestern University. He graduated from Harvard College with an A.B. in social studies and from the University of Cambridge with an M.Phil. in philosophy and received his M.D. from Harvard Medical School. After graduation from medical school, Dr. Hauser completed his residency in primary care internal medicine at the Brigham and Women's Hospital in 1998 and completed the Robert Wood Johnson Clinical Scholars Program and a fellowship in clinical medical ethics at the University of Chicago in 2001. At Harvard, the University of Chicago, the University of Illinois at Chicago, and Northwestern University, he has helped to develop successful courses in end-of-life care, medical humanism, and research ethics. His research and educational interests are in understanding the experiences of family caregivers in palliative care, developing novel teaching innovations, and evaluating professionalism. He currently chairs the professionalism competency committee at Northwestern. Clinically, he practices in the Palliative Care and Home Hospice Program at Northwestern Memorial Hospital. In professional organizations for palliative care physicians, internists, and bioethicists, Dr. Hauser has held leadership roles in palliative care and ethics, including recent co-chairman for the Ethics and Humanism workshop selection committee of the Society for General Internal Medicine, co-chairman for the program committee of the American Society of Bioethics and Humanities, and member of the ethics committee for the American Academy of Hospice and Palliative Medicine. He was also recent co-chair for an NIH study section on research ethics.

Joseph E. Kelley, M.D. (U.S. Air Force Major General, retired), is the Deputy Assistant Secretary of Defense for Clinical and Program Policy. Prior to this appointment, Dr. Kelley served as Joint Staff Surgeon, the Pentagon, Washington, DC. He served as the chief medical adviser to the Chairman of the Joint Chiefs of Staff, providing advice to the Chairman, the Joint Staff, and combatant commanders. Dr. Kelley has served as the U.S. delegate to the NATO Council of Medical Directors and served on the congressionally directed Future of Military Health Care Task Force. Dr. Kelley graduated from the U.S. Air Force Academy and received his M.D. from Rush University Medical School. He completed his residency in general surgery at David Grant Medical Center, Travis AFB, California, in combination with the University of California, Davis. He served as Chief of General Surgery at Nellis AFB and at Misawa Air Base, Japan, as Chief of Hospital Services, Chief of Surgery, and interim Chief of Aerospace Medicine. In 1986 General Kelley was reassigned as Commander of the 90th Strategic Hospital, Francis E. Warren AFB. He commanded the Ehrling Berquist Hospital at Offutt AFB, Nebraska, served as Chief of Medical Resources in the Office of the Surgeon General, and was Command Surgeon for Pacific Air Forces. He then served as Commander of the Wright-Patterson Medical Center, Wright-Patterson AFB, Ohio, and concomitantly as Assistant Dean for Government Services at the Wright State University School of Medicine. Prior to assuming the Joint Staff Surgeon position, the general was Assistant Surgeon General for Healthcare Operations, Office of the Surgeon General. General Kelley is board certified by the American Board of Surgery and is a Fellow of the American College of Surgeons.

David Ozar, Ph.D., is Professor and Co-Director of Graduate Studies in Health Care Ethics in the Department of Philosophy at Loyola University of Chicago and from 1993 to 2006 was Director of Loyola's Center for Ethics. In addition, he is Adjunct Professor of Medical Humanities in

Loyola's Stritch School of Medicine, where he has served as Acting Director of Medical Humanities. He earned his B.A. and M.A. degrees from Loyola and received his Ph.D. in philosophy from Yale University in 1974. In addition to his work at Loyola, Dr. Ozar is Associate Director of the Medical Ethics Program, a member of the Institutional Ethics Committee, and consulting ethicist at Evanston Hospital in Evanston, Illinois. He has served on the Research Review Committee of the Chicago Department of Health and is currently a member of the Executive Committee of the Chicago Region Advance Care Planning Coalition. He was the founder and first President of the American Society for Dental Ethics and has held offices in the Society for Health and Human Values, the American Philosophical Association, and other professional organizations. Dr. Ozar has published numerous articles in professional journals and books. He coedited *Philosophical Issues in Human Rights: Theories and Applications* (Random House, 1985) and, with co-author David Sokol, D.D.S., published *Dental Ethics at Chairside: Professional Principles and Practical Applications,* 2nd edition (Georgetown University Press, 2002).

Hernan Reyes, M.D., is a physician, originally trained in OB/GYN, who has been working with the International Committee of the Red Cross since 1982. His particular interest in humanitarian work has always been health issues in detention and he has visited prisoners in over 50 countries. He specializes in a series of issues, all related to health or "hazards" to health. He has published on torture and ill-treatment, tuberculosis in prisons, ethical issues such as hunger strikes and dual loyalties, HIV in prisons, and many other topics.

Elspeth Cameron Ritchie, M.D., M.P.H., is a Colonel in the U.S. Army and holds a master's degree in public health and a medical degree. She trained at Harvard University, George Washington University, Walter Reed Army Medical Center, and the Uniformed Services University of the Health Sciences, where she is an associate professor of psychiatry. Her assignments and other missions have taken her to Iraq, Israel, Korea, Somalia, and Vietnam. She brings a unique public health approach to the management of disaster and combat mental health issues and is internationally renowned as an expert on the subject. She also has published numerous articles on forensic, disaster, and military operational psychiatry. Dr. Ritchie recently completed tours as the psychiatry consultant to the U.S. Army Surgeon General and the Proponency Director of Behavioral Health and is now the Medical Director, Strategic Communication, Army Medical Department.

Leonard S. Rubenstein, J.D., is President of Physicians for Human Rights (PHR), an organization that mobilizes the health professions to advance human rights. Prior to coming to PHR, he directed the Bazelon Center for Mental Health Law, which advocates for rights and services for people with mental disabilities. A graduate of Harvard Law School and Wesleyan University, Mr. Rubenstein has spent 30 years engaged in investigation, scholarship, and advocacy relating to human rights; health and medical ethics domestically and internationally; and questions relating to medical ethics and human rights, including the role of health professionals in detainee operations. He was project leader for an international working group on the problem of dual loyalty and human rights in health professional practice, which produced the report *Dual Loyalty and Human Rights in Health Professional Practice: Proposed Guidelines and Institutional Mechanisms,* and has written extensively on questions of medical ethics and human rights, both for scholarly publications and in major media such as *The New York Times*, *Washington Post*, and *Boston Globe*. Mr. Rubenstein is a member of the Council of Foreign Relations and the Committee on Scientific Freedom and Responsibility of the American Association for the Advancement of Science. He serves on the Board of Directors of the International Federation of Health and Human Rights Organizations and the Governing Council of the American Public Health Association. He has served as an adjunct professor at Georgetown University Law School and lectures regularly at Harvard Medical School. He is the recipient of numerous awards, including the Congressional Minority Caucuses' Healthcare Hero Award; the United Nations Association of the National Capital Area's Louis B. Sohn Award; the Physicians Forum Edward K. Barsky Award; the National Mental Health Association's Mission Award; and the Political Asylum Representation Project's Outstanding Achievement Award.

Kenneth W. Schor, D.O., M.P.H., is currently an Assistant Professor in the Department of Preventive Medicine and Biometrics, Uniformed Services University of the Health Sciences (USUHS), Bethesda, Maryland, and also serves as Associate Program Director, National Capital Consortium, General Preventive Medicine Residency. Dr. Schor has over 26 years of active duty service with the U.S. Navy Medical Corps. He received his doctor of osteopathic medicine (DO) degree from the Philadelphia College of Osteopathic Medicine; is a Distinguished Graduate of the National Defense University's Industrial College of the Armed Forces; and received a master of public health (MPH) degree from USUHS. His graduate medical education includes completion of a family practice residency at Naval Hospital Jacksonville Florida, and completion of a general preventive medicine residency at USUHS. He is a Diplomate of the American Board of Preventive Medicine. Dr. Schor is the USUHS Course Director for "Joint Medical Operations and Humanitarian Assistance" and Course Director for "Public Health Issues of Disasters in Developing Countries." A pertinent collateral duty involves serving as Mission Director of an initiative for providing continuing health education (CHE) aboard Navy hospital ships. In support of the CHE mission, he was deployed July–August 2008 aboard the USNS *Mercy* as it conducted humanitarian assistance operations in the western Pacific for operation Pacific Partnership 2008.

Jack Smith, M.D., is the Director for Clinical and Program Policy Integration in the Office of the Assistant Secretary of Defense (Health Affairs). Dr. Smith's responsibilities include providing medical information, policy formulation, clinical program oversight, and consultation to senior Defense officials, congressional committees, and other government agencies. His office also provides oversight and guidance for clinical quality, patient safety, and medical management programs in the Military Health System (MHS). Dr. Smith is a graduate of the University of Virginia School of Medicine and holds a master of medical management degree from Tulane University. He served more than 30 years in the U.S. Navy and retired in 2005. He is a board-certified family physician with more than 15 years of executive medicine experience including Command of Naval Hospital, Yokosuka, Japan, and service as Group Surgeon for Second Force Service Support Group, Fleet Marine Force, Atlantic. He has been involved in a number of operational and humanitarian operations over the course of his career, including Haitian and Cuban migrant operations in Guantanamo Bay, Cuba, where he served as the Joint Task Force Surgeon in 1994, and more recently provision of support for medical-sector reconstruction projects in Afghanistan and Iraq. He is currently a leader in the MHS in strategic planning, patient safety initiatives, quality improvement, and support for wounded warriors. Dr. Smith is a Certified Physician Executive of the American College of Physician Executives, a Fellow of the American College of

Healthcare Executives, a Fellow of the American Academy of Family Physicians, and a member of a number of other professional associations.

Kurt Spindler, M.D., is Professor and Vice Chairman of the Department of Orthopaedics and Rehabilitation at Vanderbilt University School of Medicine, Director of the Vanderbilt Sports Medicine Center and the Orthopaedic Patient Care Center, and Head Team Physician for Vanderbilt University's NCAA Division I varsity athletes. He completed medical school and an orthopedic residency, including one year of basic research training, at the University of Pennsylvania. He then completed a one-year orthopedic sports medicine fellowship at the Cleveland Clinic Foundation in 1991. His practice and clinical research include prospective long-term follow-up of anterior cruciate ligament reconstructions, and he initiated the Multicenter Orthopedic Outcomes Network in 2001. Dr. Spindler is an active member of numerous regional, national, and international orthopedic and sports medicine professional organizations. He is a board member of the American Orthopedic Society for Sports Medicine (AOSSM) and Chairman of NFL Charities Grant Review Committee. His educational activities include co-chairmanship of the Advanced Team Physician Course of the AOSSM in 2000–2002 and the Complex Knee Course of the AAOS in 2002 and 2003, co-editor of *Sports Medicine Digest*, and participation on the editorial board and in the review of articles for several scientific journals.

Mahmud Thamer, M.D. M.P.H., is Assistant Professor of Medicine (retired) at Johns Hopkins University. Born in Iraq and sent after high school on a scholarship to study medicine in the United States, Dr. Thamer studied pre-med at the University of California at Berkeley and medicine at Harvard Medical School. He completed his residency and fellowship in medicine at the Johns Hopkins Bayview Medical Center and received his master of public health degree from the Johns Hopkins School of Hygiene and Public Health. Dr. Thamer returned to Iraq as a member of the Faculty of Medicine at the Baghdad Medical School and remained there for 10 years until the takeover by the Baath party. In Iraq he conducted clinical and epidemiologic studies on rheumatic heart disease, acute and chronic renal disease, and cholera. He returned to the United States as a member of the full-time faculty at the Johns Hopkins University, working in the fields of cardiac rehabilitation, cardiac consultation, and non-invasive cardiac assessment. After the overthrow of the Iraqi government in 2003, Dr. Thamer returned to Iraq for six months to serve as an adviser to the Iraqi Minister of Health on medical schools and medical education. Since retirement, he remains keenly interested in monitoring developments in Iraq and in the broader areas of Islamic-Arabic-Western understanding and dialogue.

PLANNING COMMITTEE MEMBERS

James F. Childress, Ph.D. (*Chair*), is the John Allen Hollingsworth Professor of Ethics and Professor of Medical Education at the University of Virginia (UVA), where he teaches in the Department of Religious Studies and directs the Institute for Practical Ethics and Public Life. He served as Chair of the Department of Religious Studies, 1972–1975 and 1986–1994; as Principal of UVA's Monroe Hill College from 1988 to 1991; and as Co-Director of the Virginia Health Policy Center from 1991 to 1999. In 1990 he was named Professor of the Year in the state of Virginia by the Council for the Advancement and Support of Education, and in 2002 he received the University of Virginia's highest honor—the Thomas Jefferson Award. Dr. Childress was Vice Chair of the National Task Force on Organ Transplantation, and he has also served on the Board of Directors of the United Network for Organ Sharing (UNOS), the UNOS Ethics Committee, the Recombinant DNA Advisory Committee, the Human Gene Therapy Subcommittee, the Biomedical Ethics Advisory Committee, and several Data and Safety Monitoring Boards for NIH clinical trials. He was a member of the presidentially appointed National Bioethics Advisory Commission from 1996 to 2001. Dr. Childress is a member of the Institute of Medicine and a fellow of the American Academy of Arts and Sciences. He is also a fellow of the Hastings Center. He received his B.A. from Guilford College, his B.D. from Yale Divinity School, and his M.A. and Ph.D. from Yale University. Dr. Childress chaired the IOM Committee on Increasing Rates of Organ Donation, co-chaired the NRC Subcommittee on Use of Third Party Toxicity Research with Human Test Subjects, and has served as a member of the IOM Committee on Establishing a National Cord Blood Stem Cell Bank Program and the Committee on Assessing Genetic Risks: Issues and Implications for Health. He currently serves as a member of the IOM Board on Health Sciences Policy and the IOM Committee on Conflicts of Interest in Medical Research, Education, and Practice.

Scott Allen, M.D., is the co-director of the Center for Prisoner Health and Human Rights at Brown University and Clinical Assistant Professor of Medicine at the Alpert Medical School. Dr. Allen has worked in the correctional field for the past decade, including seven years as a full-time physician at the Rhode Island Department of Corrections, including three as Medical Program Director (2001–2004). He has spoken and written about a number of correctional health and human rights issues, including hepatitis C in prisons and the obligations of health professionals in protecting the human rights of inmate patients. He has served as a court-appointed expert to the federal courts in prison health cases. He is a former Medicine as a Profession Fellow and currently an adviser for Physicians for Human Rights in Cambridge, Massachusetts, and an attending medical physician for an inpatient psychiatric ward at Eleanor Slater Hospital in Cranston, Rhode Island.

Paul S. Appelbaum, M.D., is the Elizabeth K. Dollard Professor of Psychiatry, Medicine, and Law and Director, Division of Psychiatry, Law, and Ethics, Department of Psychiatry, College of Physicians and Surgeons of Columbia University. Dr. Appelbaum is Past President of the American Psychiatric Association, the American Academy of Psychiatry and the Law, and the Massachusetts Psychiatric Society and serves as Chair of the Council on Psychiatry and Law for the American Psychiatric Association. He was previously Chair of the Commission on Judicial Action for the American Psychiatric Association and a member of the MacArthur Foundation Research Network on Mental Health and the Law. He is currently a member of the MacArthur Foundation Network on Mandatory Outpatient Treatment. He was the Fritz Redlich Fellow at the Center for Advanced Study in the Behavioral Sciences and has been elected to the Institute of Medicine of the National Academy of Sciences. Dr. Appelbaum is a graduate of Columbia College, received his M.D. from Harvard Medical School, and completed his residency in psychiatry at the Massachusetts Mental Health Center in Boston. He is a member of the workshop planning committee and also currently serves on the IOM Committee on Health Research and the Privacy of Health Information.

Thomas E. Beam, M.D., retired from the U.S. Army in 2001 after 30 years of service as a general surgeon. He held several clinical positions, including Assistant Chief, Department of Surgery, during his time at Walter Reed Army Medical Center. While he was on active duty, he directed the Borden Institute, Office of the Surgeon General, producing the

Textbook of Military Medicine series and other special projects for the Army Surgeon General. He produced the *Textbook of Military Medical Ethics* for that series. He was the consultant to the Army Surgeon General in medical ethics. He represented the Army on the Tri-Service Ethics Consultants Board and continues to serve with this group. Dr. Beam was also the Chairman, Hospital Ethics Committee, for the Walter Reed Army Medical Center for almost 10 years and continues to work with this committee. He has done extensive work in ethics education, ethics consultation, and policy formation in military medical ethics. He is a Fellow of The Center for Bioethics and Human Dignity and member of the Christian Medical and Dental Associations, currently serving on their Ethics Commission. Dr. Beam received his B.A. summa cum laude from Western Maryland College and his M.D. from the University of Virginia. He served a residency in general surgery at Walter Reed Army Medical Center and received the Erskine Award as outstanding resident at Walter Reed for 1980. He is an Assistant Professor of Surgery in the Uniformed Services University of the Health Sciences and a diplomat of the American Board of Surgery and fellow in the American College of Surgery.

Richard J. Bonnie, LL.B., is the Harrison Foundation Professor of Medicine and Law, Professor of Psychiatry and Neurobehavioral Sciences, and Director of the Institute of Law, Psychiatry, and Public Policy at the University of Virginia. He teaches and writes about criminal law, bioethics, and public policies relating to mental health, substance abuse, aging, and public health. Among many other positions, he has been Associate Director of the National Commission on Marihuana and Drug Abuse, Secretary of the first National Advisory Council on Drug Abuse, chair of Virginia's State Human Rights Committee responsible for protecting rights of persons with mental disabilities, and chief adviser for the ABA Criminal Justice Mental Health Standards Project. He is currently chairing a Commission on Mental Health Law Reform at the request of the Chief Justice of Virginia. Professor Bonnie has served as an adviser to the American Psychiatric Association Council on Psychiatry and Law since 1979, received the APA's Isaac Ray Award in 1998 for contributions to forensic psychiatry, and was awarded a special presidential commendation in 2003 for his contributions to American psychiatry. He has also served on the MacArthur Foundation Research Network on Mental Health and the Law. Professor Bonnie is a member of the Institute of Medicine, has chaired numerous Academy studies on subjects ranging from elder mistreatment to underage drinking, and just completed chairing a major IOM study on tobacco policy. He received the Yarmolinsky Medal in 2002 for his contributions to the IOM and the National Academies. In 2007 Professor Bonnie received the University of Virginia's highest honor, the Thomas Jefferson Award.

Lonnie Bristow, M.D., is a former President of the American Medical Association, after earlier serving as Vice Chair and Chair of the AMA's Board of Trustees. Dr. Bristow has written and lectured extensively on medical science as well as socioeconomic and ethical issues related to medicine. He is a board-certified internist who received his M.D. from New York University College of Medicine. He is a member of the Institute of Medicine and was a member of its Quality of Health Care in America Committee, which in 1999 and 2001, respectively, authored the widely read reports *To Err Is Human* and *Crossing the Quality Chasm*. He chaired the IOM Committee on Strategies for Increasing the Diversity of the U.S. Health Care Workforce, which issued its report, *In the Nation's Compelling Interest: Ensuring Diversity in the Health Care Workforce*, in 2004. In 2005 the IOM appointed Dr. Bristow to chair a committee formed in response to our government's request to ascertain what improvements are needed, specifically from the medical perspective, in meeting our nation's responsibilities to its disabled veterans. The committee's 2007 report, *A 21st Century System for Evaluating Veteran's Disability Benefits*, with its recommendations, is under consideration by Congress for legislative action. Dr. Bristow's research interests and expertise are eclectic and, over the decades, his writings have included papers on medical ethics, socialized medicine as practiced in Great Britain and Canada, health care financing in America, professional liability insurance problems, sickle cell anemia, and coronary care unit utilization. Dr. Bristow, by presidential appointment, served from 1996 to 2001 as Chair of the Board of Regents of the Uniformed Services University of the Health Sciences. He recently retired from private practice but continues his other activities as a professional consultant.

Linda Emanuel, M.D., Ph.D., is the Buehler Professor of Geriatric Medicine and Director of the Buehler Center on Aging, Health & Society at Northwestern's Feinberg School of Medicine. She is the founder and principal of the national Education in Palliative and End-of-life Care (EPEC) Project and the Patient Safety Education Project (PSEP). She is also a professor at the Kellogg School of Management at Northwestern University, where she works on organizational ethics and on economic modeling of and resilience options against the illness–poverty trap. Prior to joining Northwestern University, Dr. Emanuel was Vice President of Ethics Standards and Head of the Institute for Ethics at the American Medical Association. Until 1996 Dr. Emanuel was the Assistant Director, Division of Medical Ethics, and until 1998 the Glessner Lee Associate Professor of Medical Ethics at Harvard Medical School. She has published and lectured extensively on clinical ethics, including end-of-life care, the patient–physician relationship, academic integrity, accountability, organizational ethics, and professionalism. Dr. Emanuel was trained at Cambridge University, University College London, Oxford University, Harvard Medical School, and Harvard University. She is a board-certified general internist with board-level specialization in palliative care, fellowship training in public health research methodology, and fellowship training in professional ethics. Prior to her clinical career, Dr. Emanuel was a research neurophysiologist, in which field she earned her Ph.D.

Edmund Howe, M.D., J.D., is a Professor of psychiatry at the F. Edward Hebert School of Medicine of the Uniformed Services University of the Health Sciences (USUHS) in Bethesda, Maryland, and is Director of the Programs in Ethics. He is a Senior Scientist at the Center for the Study of Traumatic Stress, USUHS, and the founding Editor-in-Chief of the *Journal of Clinical Ethics.* Dr. Howe did his undergraduate studies at Yale University and received his M.D. from Columbia School of Medicine in 1970. He did his rotating internship at Harlem Hospital in New York and attended law school at Rutgers University and Catholic University in Washington, DC, receiving his J.D. in 1976. Dr. Howe did his psychiatric residency at Walter Reed Army Medical Center, Washington, DC, from 1973 to 1976. Dr. Howe serves on the ethics committees at the National Naval Medical Center, the Walter Reed Army Medical Center, and the Montgomery Hospice Association. He chairs the institutional review board at USUHS. Dr. Howe has published extensively on ethical aspects of military medicine and international health law, including serving as co-editor of the textbook *Military Medical Ethics*.

Sandral Hullett, M.D., M.P.H., is Chief Executive Officer and Medical Director of Cooper Green Hospital in Birmingham, Alabama. She earned her undergraduate degree in biology at Alabama A&M University, her medical degree from the Medical College of Pennsylvania, and her master's in public health from the University of Alabama at Birmingham. She completed her residency in family practice and has focused her work on rural health care, including health care planning and delivery to the underinsured and poor. Dr. Hullett was honored with the National Rural Health Association's Rural Practitioner of the Year Award in 1988, the National Association of Community Health Centers' Clinical Recognition Award for Education and Training in 1993, Leadership Alabama's Distinguished Leadership Award in 1996, and the National Black Churches Family Council's Rural Leadership Image Award in 1998. Dr. Hullett served for 19 years on the Board of Trustees of the University of Alabama. She was elected to IOM membership in 1995. Dr. Hullett has served on the IOM Committee on Environmental Justice and the IOM Committee on the Changing Market, Managed Care, and the Future Viability of Safety Net Providers. She currently serves on the National Academies' Committee on Human Rights.

M. E. Bonnie Rogers, Dr.P.H., COHN-S, FAAN, is an Associate Professor of Nursing and Public Health and Director of the North Carolina Occupational Safety and Health Education and Research Center and the Occupational Health Nursing Program at the University of North Carolina, School of Public Health, Chapel Hill. Dr. Rogers received her diploma in nursing from the Washington Hospital Center School of Nursing, Washington, DC; her baccalaureate in nursing from George Mason University, School of Nursing, Fairfax, Virginia; and her master of public health degree and doctorate in public health from the Johns Hopkins University School of Hygiene and Public Health. Dr. Rogers was a visiting ethics scholar at the Hastings Center in New York and is an ethics consultant. She is certified in occupational health nursing and as a legal nurse consultant and is a Fellow in the American Academy of Nursing and the American Association of Occupational Health Nurses. Dr. Rogers serves as Chairperson of the NIOSH National Occupational Research Agenda Liaison Committee and is a member of the American College of Occupational and Environmental Medicine Ethics Committee. She has served on numerous Institute of Medicine committees including Nursing, Health and the Environment and the Committee to Assess Training Needs for Occupational Safety and Health Personnel in the United States. Dr. Rogers is Past President of the American Association of Occupational Health Nurses.

Adviser to the Planning Committee

Elena Ottolenghi Nightingale, M.D., Ph.D., is a Scholar-in-Residence at the Institute of Medicine of the National Academy of Sciences and Adjunct Professor of Pediatrics at both Georgetown University Medical Center and George Washington University Medical Center. For more than 11 years she was Special Adviser to the President and Senior Program Officer at Carnegie Corporation of New York and lecturer in social medicine at Harvard University. She retired from both positions at the end of 1994. Dr. Nightingale earned an A.B. degree in zoology, summa cum laude, from Barnard College of Columbia University, a Ph.D. in microbial genetics from the Rockefeller University, and an M.D. from New York University School of Medicine. With Eric Stover, she co-edited *The Breaking of Bodies and Minds: Torture, Psychiatric Abuse and the Health Professions*, published in 1985, one of the earliest efforts to discuss this topic. She has also authored numerous book chapters and articles on microbial genetics, health (particularly child and adolescent health and well-being and health promotion and disease prevention), health policy, and human rights. Dr. Nightingale continues to be active in the protection of human rights, particularly those of children. Currently she serves on the Advisory Committee of the Children's Rights Division of Human Rights Watch. Dr. Nightingale is a member of the Institute of Medicine of the National Academy of Sciences. In her role as Scholar-in-Residence, Dr. Nightingale serves as adviser to the President and Executive Officer of the Institute of Medicine.